Erica White's

Beat Candida Cookbook

*Over 300 recipes with a 4-point plan
for attacking candidiasis*

Erica White

Thorsons
An Imprint of HarperCollinsPublishers

Thorsons
An Imprint of HarperCollins*Publishers*
77–85 Fulham Palace Road
Hammersmith, London W6 8JB

The Thorsons website address is: www.thorsons.com

Published by Thorsons 1999

10 9 8 7 6 5 4 3

A catalogue record for this book
is available from the British Library

ISBN 0 7225 3856 1

Printed and bound in Great Britain by
Scotprint, Haddington, Scotland

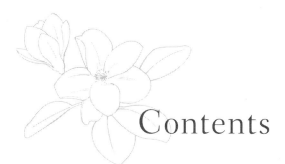

Contents

Part Three: Helpful Ideas

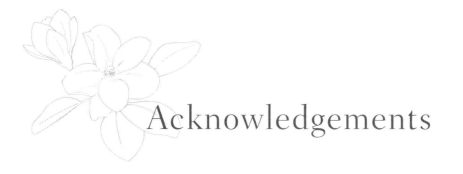

Acknowledgements

Two people played a key part in helping me to become established as a Nutrition Consultant, and I wish to thank them here.

Dr John Stirling, of BioCare Limited, Birmingham, UK, helped me to understand the role and use of caprylic acid in overcoming my own candida problems, and many times gave me the benefit of his experience as my practice started to develop.

Patrick Holford, founder of the Institute for Optimum Nutrition in London, made it possible for me to learn about the miraculous design of the human body and the role of optimum nutrition in its efficient functioning. As my tutor, he encouraged me to put my training and experience into practice, even though I was already a grandmother!

Many of my clients responded enthusiastically when I asked them to send me their favourite recipes for the first edition of this book, and many more were just as enthusiastic to contribute to this second edition eight years later. I thank them all and apologize that not every submission has been included or that they might not recognize their own version of a particular dish because many have been amalgamated or adapted. However, the ideas which came in were invaluable, and I am extremely grateful to these clients:

First edition: Helen Agarwal, Jill Bartlett, Kay Beighton, Meg Cheeseman, the late Margaret Cockerell, Yvonne Currie, Louise Davidge, Karen Davies, Nicola Doherty, Jane French, Sheila Gibson, Mandy Gilbart-Smith, Eleanor Gleadow, Valerie Grant, Barbara Graves, Angela Holmes, Lynne Mahoney, Moira McQuiggan, Heather Strachan, Valerie Sumpton, Sarah Watkins, Judi Whitehead, Rosie de Wolf, Marion Wright, Julia Yarrell.

Second edition: Jonathan Bayes, Philippa Bodien, Andrea Budd, Susan Chamberlain, Pauline Fuller, Janet Hammond, Robert Heath, Diane Highton, Colleen Jarvis, Frances Lafarge, Linda Pilgrim, Lynne Rodgers, Lindsey Stringer, Jacqui Upton, Clare Watts, Caroline West, Jennifer West, Elaine Williams, Natalie Williams, Marion Wright.

My special thanks go to my daughter, Emma Cockrell, who is a far more gifted cook than I am and who checked, advised, suggested, generally put me straight, and managed in her very busy life to experiment with various recipes. Emma herself had a long personal experience of candida and this, combined with an inspirational approach towards wholefood cookery and challenging diets, has given her an expertise coveted by many – especially me!

And lastly I thank my husband, Robin, who gave up his own career to throw himself into the administration of our Nutrition Consultancy and mastermind the computerization of the calculations for our reports. Many wives envy the way in which my husband sacrificed his own work in order to work with me, but I know that in fact he is more fulfilled than ever before. My main cause for gratitude is that he stood by me, as did our three children, through all the many years when candida, the unknown enemy, caused me so much suffering and distress. I was not aware of just how unusual and special that was until I came across marriages which had been tossed on the heap by candida. So, after 40 years of very happy marriage, all I can say is thank you.

Introduction

In 1988, at the age of 53, I discovered a way of beating the candida overgrowth which had been the cause of a lifetime of ill health. Within a few months I had started a course of training to become a qualified Nutrition Consultant. By 1991, it was clear that with the combination of my experience and my training, I was able to help an enormous number of people who were suffering as I had, and to help them even further I wrote the *Beat Candida Cookbook*. It took months of hard work to put it together and type it on an ancient, huge word processor. When it was finished, we photocopied 50 sets and put acetate covers on them with a borrowed comb-binding machine.

The first 50 sets disappeared before we knew it so we photocopied another hundred, and they continued to go as fast as we could prepare them. It became so time-consuming that we paid someone else to do the copying, but before long it was too much for one person so we decided to have it professionally printed – keeping the same format since it was evidently so popular – and to set up our own publishing company. Other nutritionists and some stores began to stock it for their clients and customers, and we soon had to ask our printer for two more reprints. We had no distribution network apart from the obviously powerful word-of-mouth which led to sales of over 11,000 copies.

I was approached by a Norwegian publishing company, Ex Libris, for my permission to produce a Norwegian translation of the book, which I gladly gave. Now I have been approached by Thorsons to produce an updated English edition. This is an offer I am delighted to accept, because first of all I know that the book needs to contain some of the additional knowledge I have acquired in the eight years since I first wrote it.

Secondly, I know that there is an enormous number of people, worldwide, who are struggling with yeast infection and who need the help which a wider distribution of this book can bring. If you are one of them, I pray that this updated, enlarged and attractive new edition of my *Beat Candida Cookbook* will do as much and more for you as the previous, home-spun edition was able to do for thousands of earlier readers. Enjoy the book, enjoy the food, be encouraged – and get well!

Erica White
July 1999

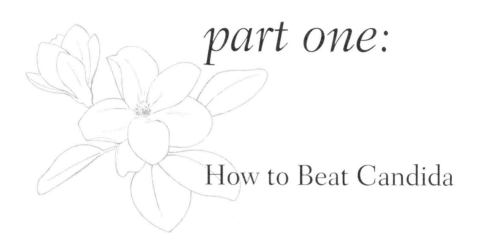

part one:

How to Beat Candida

Chapter 1

About Candida Albicans

My guess is that you are probably reading this book because you already know, or at least strongly suspect, that you are suffering from yeast-related health problems – the effects of an overgrowth of Candida albicans – and that you are looking for ways to overcome them. On the other hand, it may be that you have heard something about Candida albicans and are just wondering whether this might be the cause of your own health problems.

This book does not set out to be a scientific textbook on the subject; I leave that to other authors. It is basically what its title implies – a collection of recipes to help you enjoy an anti-candida diet. However, diet alone will not beat candida; it is just one part of the necessary programme. So, first of all, if you are uncertain as to whether candida might be the cause of your ill-health, I would like to help you clarify the situation by explaining a little more about it. Then, if you are still uncertain that your problems do have a yeast connection but medical explorations have left you with no other explanation, I suggest that you complete the simple score sheet at the back of the book. This should leave you in little doubt, one way or the other. If your candida score is higher than it should be, I would like to help you rediscover your health by describing the method which worked first of all for me, and which I have since recommended to clients in my nutritional practice for several years. In order to explain the reasons behind the recommendations, I need to give you a very simple outline of what yeast infection is all about and how it is thought to cause so many different health problems.

Let me start by giving you some idea of just how many health problems might be associated with an overgrowth of Candida albicans, the condition known as yeast infection or candidiasis.

Conditions of the skin: athlete's foot, ringworm, psoriasis, eczema, rashes, itching, easy bruising, acne, fungal nail conditions.

Conditions of the digestive tract: abdominal pain, constipation or diarrhoea, irritable bowel syndrome, bloating, belching, intestinal gas, indigestion or heartburn, mucus in stools, rash or blisters in the mouth (oral thrush), painful oesophagus, rectal irritation, food sensitivity or intolerance, dry mouth or throat, bad breath.

Conditions of the reproductive system: vaginal burning, irritation or discharge (thrush), endometriosis, infertility, period pains, menstrual irregularities, premenstrual tension, breast tenderness, loss of sexual feeling. In men: impotence, prostatitis.

Conditions of the urinary tract: frequency, burning, urgency.

Conditions of eyes, ears, nose, throat and chest: nasal congestion, post-nasal drip (catarrh or mucus running down back of throat), itchy nose, sore throat, laryngitis, loss of voice, cough, recurrent bronchitis, pain or tightness in the chest, wheezing, shortness of breath, asthma, spots in front of eyes, erratic vision, burning or watering eyes, recurrent infections in ears, fluid in ears, ear pain, deafness, sinusitis, dizziness, loss of balance.

Conditions of joints, muscles and nervous system: muscle aches, muscle weakness, paralysis, painful joints, swollen joints, numbness, burning or tingling.

Conditions affecting the mind, as well as the body: fatigue, lethargy, feeling drained, depression, poor memory, feeling 'spacey' or 'unreal', inability to make decisions, attacks of anxiety or crying, panic, drowsiness, irritability, jitteriness, lack of co-ordination, inability to concentrate, mood swings, pressure above the ears, a feeling of the head swelling, insomnia.

Poor circulation: cold hands and feet, general chilliness.

Shakiness or irritability when hungry.

Body odour which is not relieved by washing.

There are even further symptoms besides these and, if you add them to a weakened immune system and therefore an increased tendency to allergy and a decreased resistance to infection, you have some idea of how widespread and how devastating the effects of candida can be – so it's very good to know that we have a way of beating it!

There may be other problems which will be uncovered along the way, but most of these can be dealt with more easily once the candida has been brought under control. For instance, if food allergy is part of your picture, it is probably due to the fact that candida has made your intestinal wall porous. This means that minute particles of food are able to escape into your bloodstream before they have been fully digested. In this form, the food is regarded by the immune system as a foe rather than a friend, so it mounts an attack and you get an unpleasant reaction. Once the candida is under control, it is possible to help the intestinal wall to heal so that it is no longer porous, which means that it is also possible to overcome the vast majority of food sensitivities.

So, what exactly *is* Candida albicans, and how does it manage to create so many problems in our bodies?

Let's start at the beginning. In our intestines, we each carry about four pounds in weight of live micro-organisms. That's quite a load! When we are healthy, these microbes are divided into about 80 per cent 'good guys' and 20 per cent 'bad guys' – although in fact the bad guys are not harmful provided they stay in their 20-per-cent boundary. One of these potential bad guys is a common yeast called Candida albicans which, like the others, lives in each one of us but causes no problems as long as it is kept firmly within its boundary lines. Unfortunately, several things are happening in this day and age which encourage it to grow stronger and to spread. This situation of overgrowth causes all the trouble because, having started life as a spore, thriving candida changes into a fungal form, with roots called mycelia which can penetrate the tissues of the body.

The first major cause of the problem is the amount of sugar we all eat. If you have ever made your own bread or wine, you will know that sugar is necessary to activate the yeast. In so-called civilized countries today, we eat so much sugar that each person is reckoned to consume roughly his own body-weight in sugar every year, whereas 100 years ago we ate only about 10 pounds of sugar each in a year! In fact, our bodies need no added sugar at all for energy or health, apart from the natural sugars found in fruits, vegetables and grains, so this vast amount of surplus sugar is encouraging the yeast in our bodies to thrive, among many other harmful effects.

How do we manage to eat such great quantities of sugar? Well, besides putting it in our coffee and tea, we eat it in biscuits, cakes, ice-creams, sweets, cereals, puddings and pies and in many other foods which come in packets, tins, bottles and jars. Often, we don't even suspect that it's there! It's in cans of beans and bottles of ketchup, in many frozen vegetables, in most breakfast cereals (which we then smother with more!) and in bottles of fizzy drink; one well-known brand has the equivalent of 22 spoons of sugar in every bottle.

Added to this heavy intake of sugar, we need to realize that refined grains (like white flour used for bread, cakes and biscuits, and also white rice and cornflour/cornstarch) turn to glucose very quickly once eaten, making the level of sugar in our blood rise even higher which, again, feeds the yeast in our bodies. You can begin to see how well we look after our resident candida!

Another cause of the problem which has come about in recent years is the use – and often, it has to be said, the over-use – of antibiotics. These powerful antibacterial drugs – welcome life-savers in emergency situations – unfortunately have the effect of destroying the beneficial bacteria in our intestines as well as those that are making us ill. As the good guys are depleted, more space is created for thriving candida, and so it claims more ground. When, for example, antibiotics are given for months on end (and sometimes even years) to treat acne, or when they are given several times in a year to treat a recurrent sore throat, the knock-on effect on the balance of our intestinal bacteria is devastating. Very often, acne and recurrent infections have been caused by candida in the first place, so taking antibiotics simply makes matters worse. Apart from the antibiotics we are prescribed, there are residues in the meat which we eat and the milk which we drink, because animals are treated with them as a preventative against disease. To avoid this, you need either to become a strict vegetarian or else to eat meat from animals which have been organically reared.

Other types of medication also have the capacity to destroy our friendly bacteria. Non-steroidal anti-inflammatory drugs (NSAIDs), available over the counter, are used extremely widely for period pain, back ache and other painful conditions, and these, just like antibiotics, prepare the way for candida to move in and gain more ground.

Another main cause of yeast infection is the use of steroid treatments. Sufferers of hayfever and asthma who regularly use steroid sprays or inhalers are actually weakening their immune systems even further, because although in the short-term steroids have a potent anti-inflammatory effect, in the long-term they also have an acknowledged immuno-suppressant effect. An increasingly weakened immune system will be less and less able to hold back invading bad guys, including candida, and many asthma sufferers have thrush in their mouths, throats and oesophagus which has been caused by their steroid puffers. Similarly, many fungal skin conditions are mistakenly treated with steroid creams which not only are absorbed into the body and weaken the immune system, but which also make the situation increasingly chronic, even though they might well have short-term benefits in reducing pain, inflammation, irritation and danger.

I need to say here that it could be extremely dangerous for you to stop taking any steroid medication without first discussing the situation with your doctor and asking if a viable alternative can be prescribed. If your doctor is concerned that your asthma, for example, still requires the help of steroids, start on your nutritional programme for a few months and then ask your doctor to check you over again; there could then well be encouraging improvements which would enable your medical practitioner to allow you a trial period without the steroid treatment.

It is sadly not often realized that any type of hormone treatment, including HRT for menopausal problems and also the contraceptive pill, is in fact a form of steroid treatment which will suppress the immune system in just the same way as other steroids, thus allowing candida to gain more of a hold.

It is not unusual to come across a young woman who is riddled with candida and has unknowingly been doing everything possible to encourage the situation! She might have been prescribed the Pill since her early teens to help with difficult periods and she might also have been on long-term antibiotics for stubborn acne – caused initially by a high-sugar diet and other nutritional imbalances but then encouraged by the Pill to become a fungal skin condition! In fact, so many people are suffering because of these three major factors – hormone or steroid treatments, antibiotics and a high-sugar diet, that there is virtually an epidemic of candida-related problems, and yet it largely goes unrecognized.

Within the female body, hormones and candida very strongly interact. Changes in hormone levels throughout the menstrual cycle, and also during pregnancy and at the menopause, greatly encourage candida activity. For this reason, and also probably due to the fact that yeast thrives in warm, dark, moist places, more women than men are afflicted with candida problems. That is not to say that men don't have them; I see an increasing number of men in my practice and many are extremely ill. Usually, it is a man's digestive tract which suffers most, giving rise to intestinal gas and irritable bowel syndrome, but he also might suffer from depression and, just as with a woman, an overgrowth of candida plays havoc with his immune system.

Even small children don't escape; if a mother has thrush when she gives birth, candida will be the first microbe to enter the baby's previously sterile gastro-intestinal tract. Since the hormonal influence means that thrush is very frequently present during pregnancy (especially if the mother had previously taken the Pill), many babies will begin life infested with candida as a result. Breast milk contains anti-fungal properties which obviously help to establish a healthy balance of bacteria in the baby's intestines but, even so, if the baby has been infected with candida before it has a chance to suck milk, the battle has already begun. It will show itself in the baby's mouth as white patches, or it will appear as severe nappy rash. This small human being will almost certainly suffer from sleep-disrupting colic, from earache, so that grommets are inserted at an early age, and possibly from eczema. Without doubt he will suffer from the effects of a weak immune system – hayfever, asthma and constant coughs and colds, leading to poor attendance at school. By the time he has taken innumerable courses of antibiotics and used a steroid puffer and steroid creams, his immune system will be almost totally broken down and he will be in a state of chronic fatigue.

Yet another dimension needs to be added to this picture. Why is it that some people succumb to the effects of an overgrowth of candida more readily than others – even though they might be living the same lifestyle, sharing the same house and eating the same food? The answer is to do with the strength of our individual immune systems. Each one of us is unique. Not only have our bodies inherited different strengths and weaknesses but the various events of our lives have also played a part in determining what is called our 'biochemical individuality'. Some people have inherited a strong resistance to infection; others have not. Some have been breast-fed as babies; others have been bottle-fed on a cow's milk formula. Some have grown up in the comparatively pure air of the countryside; others spent their childhood surrounded by industrial pollution. Some ate large amounts of sweets and junk food as children; others had plenty of home-grown fruit and vegetables. These are pretty black-and-white contrasts, but you will probably be able to see which of the situations apply to you, and perhaps also begin to see why it is that you have health problems when others do not.

The air we now breathe is full of traces of poisonous metals – lead from petrol and cadmium from factory chimneys are just two. In addition, many of us are absorbing aluminium from antiperspirants and indigestion tablets, and most of us are absorbing traces of mercury from the amalgam fillings in our teeth – that is, those of us who have some teeth left! Our bodies were not made to cope with such a load of poisons, and our immune systems are over-worked – often to the point of exhaustion – in an attempt to keep us in what we have come to accept as 'good health', not realizing how far short it falls of the real thing. Many of us have no idea of what it feels like to be *really* healthy. With so much work to do, the struggling immune system tries to fight back at the bad guys which are taking more and more ground from the good guys in our intestines.

As the immune system grows weaker, candida grows stronger and, when it is thriving, it actually changes its shape and grows whisker-like roots so that, seen through a microscope, it looks very much like mould growing on an old loaf of bread. Once it is in this fungal form, candida is able to burrow through the wall of the intestines and enter the bloodstream, so that it is then free to travel anywhere in the body, burrowing into other tissues and setting up colonies wherever it fancies! It gets into muscles, joints, skin and mucous membranes.

(If you find this hard to believe, it has been confirmed by reputable scientists and doctors. As far back as 1984, Dr Jeffrey Bland, writing in the journal, *Preventive Medicine*, said 'The breakdown of gastrointestinal mucosa can also lead to the introduction of the candida organism into the bloodstream and it can then find its way into other tissues, resulting in far-ranging systemic effects, including soreness of joints, chest pain and skin problems.' Dr Ralph Golan, writing in *Optimal Wellness*, says, 'Wherever the yeast colonise, they cause symptoms, whether an itchy anus or vagina, diarrhoea, heart-burn or sore throat. They can also colonise the sinuses and trigger sinus, ear and eye symptoms.' And Dr William Shaw, in his book, *Biological Treatments for Autism and PDD*, says, 'It (the yeast) can invade virtually any organ of the body including the blood, the lungs, bones, kidneys, the liver, the heart, the eyes and the brain.')

Candida also releases poisons (79 have been identified) which affect the brain and nervous system. In fact, it creates havoc. And the body in which it is having such a great time is made to feel 'ill all over'.

The weakened immune system becomes even weaker, trying to fight a losing battle. The body starts to develop allergies, reacting badly to things in the environment which other people do not notice – things like pollen, dust, mould, perfume and household gas. This is in addition to the food sensitivities which develop as a result of candida causing a 'leaky gut syndrome', providing yet another problem for the weakened immune system to cope with.

For many people, the next thing to happen is that they become ill with a viral infec-tion – some type of influenza or a tummy bug, or possibly glandular fever – and they find that they cannot get over it. The illness drags on and on. They feel incredibly weak and exhausted. Eventually, hospital tests are made and sometimes a virus is found, some-times not. When it is, and a diagnosis can be given, the sufferer is reassured to know that at least his illness is something which is recognized, something with a name. But when the name is ME (Myalgic Encephalomyelitis) or CFS (Chronic Fatigue Syndrome) or PVF (Post-Viral Fatigue) or CFIDS (Chronic Fatigue and Immune Dysfunction Syndrome), the patient very often is left in despair because nobody seems to know how to help him. He has no more hope of recovery than before the diagnosis was made.

When not even a virus is found, the patient may be branded a malingerer by his doctor and so have great difficulty in claiming sickness benefits or other state support, yet he is far too weak or ill to be able to work. All these problems have to be endured besides the wide-ranging symptoms of the illness, which include chronic fatigue and muscle weakness, very often to the point of being bed-bound. It is not surprising that many relationships and marriages suffer and even fall apart under the strain. Life becomes a torment.

In my book, *M.E.: Sailing Free*, I explain how various situations or conditions place a load on the immune system, leading to a severe breakdown in health. These factors might include allergy, low blood sugar, underactive thyroid, pollution and toxicity, infec-tion and stress; but, in the many hundreds of ME sufferers I have come across in the course of my work, there has always been one common denominator – an overgrowth of the common yeast, Candida albicans! There is no doubt that candida contributes to a complete breakdown of the immune system, so that it is unable to fight off an attacking virus. In fact, when a virus has not been found, I sometimes wonder if the medical diagnosis of ME (or CFS or CFIDS) is correct, because all the symptoms which go to make up Chronic Fatigue Syndrome are indistinguishable from severe candidiasis; and in any case, in my experience, the answers to both conditions are the same.

It would, of course, be so much easier to make a diagnosis if adequate tests were available, but most of the tests which have been devised do not, in my opinion, give either the total picture or a sufficiently clear one. For instance, a stool test will not even tell you how much candida is on the intestinal wall, so it will certainly not be able to tell you how much has migrated to your painful elbow! Blood tests, swabs and breath tests all have their shortfalls (read about them in *Optimal Wellness* by Dr Ralph Golan) but possibly a urine test showing by-products of yeast in the body (discussed by Dr William Shaw in *Biological Treatments for Autism and PDD*) is the most correct and therefore the most useful. However, it is expensive and in my experience it is unnecessary in the vast majority of cases.

In my practice I use a simple questionnaire which lists many possible candida-related symptoms as well as possible predisposing factors. For many years I used the questionnaire devised by Dr William Crook in his ground-breaking book, *The Yeast Connection*, but the score sheet at the back of this book is one which I have now developed myself. Of course, each symptom on its own might be due to other causes, but the coincidence of having more than a few of these symptoms leaves little doubt that in fact they do have a common cause. One big advantage of using a questionnaire is that it provides you with a score giving an indication of the severity of the problem. This means that after a period of time you can see how much improvement has been made by watching the score come down. In my practice, I review the situation at three-month intervals and look for a continuing drop in the candida score; I can also see clearly how much candida still remains to be dealt with and decide on the best way to tackle the specific symptoms remaining.

And the good news is that it *can* be dealt with! It *is* possible to be healthy once more! It *is* possible to take loads off the immune system and strengthen it so that it functions efficiently again! And it *is* possible to bring the overgrowth of candida under control and rid the body of its effects! It isn't easy; it takes determination and perseverance, but it can be done! I speak from experience in my own life and from seeing it happen in countless other lives since.

Let me tell you my story.

Chapter 2

Candida and Me

I was born in 1935 and, right through to 1988, I battled against ill health. I was so frequently out of action that I look back and wonder how on earth we managed to bring up a family of three children.

As a child, I was always away from school with colds or 'bilious attacks', and my earliest memory is of 'feeling sore' at three years old and being sat in a bowl of warm water which smelled of antiseptic! I developed school phobia, largely because I was terrified of physical education lessons – a fear which I now believe was due to my very poor sense of balance; I dreaded having to be upside-down or turn a somersault!

As a teenager, I developed constant sinusitis and frequent bouts of influenza, both of which went on to plague me for many years to come. I also developed back problems, teeth problems, cystitis, fibrositis – you name it, I usually had it! Nothing in itself was life-threatening, but all the time there was some part of my body which was hurting and drawing attention to itself, and for much of the time I felt ill and exhausted. However, I didn't take the situation lying down and I constantly fought back, making tremendous efforts with jobs and other activities, often aware that I was actually working harder than most other people! I was tall with rosy cheeks, and it was obvious that many people thought I was simply neurotic about my health. All through my life, the attitude of people (both friends and doctors) to someone who was constantly feeling ill with no apparent cause was quite difficult to cope with.

In 1959, I married Robin, and over the next 10 years I had three babies – with horrendously sick pregnancies and other health problems all the time. After our third baby, Hannah, was born in 1969, I developed gallstones, although for six months they were not diagnosed and I was told by a hospital specialist that my terrible pains were due to post-natal depression!

Eventually, my gall-bladder was removed and I was given a bottle full of stones to take home with me. However, within a few weeks of the operation I was in a state of almost total physical collapse. Thirty years on, I am certain that my condition would now be diagnosed as ME but, in 1969, very few people – including doctors – had yet come across it. I would struggle to the corner shop, about a hundred yards away, and then have to lie on my bed for the rest of the day, utterly exhausted, aching all over, and with palpitations shaking my body. With two small children and a baby to look after, it was no joke.

After a year, my mother mentioned that a friend of hers had been having really severe asthma attacks ever since the gas supply to her house had been converted to the new North Sea gas. As our house had also been converted, she wondered whether it might be having some sort of effect on me. Robin and I found it hard to believe that ordinary domestic gas would have such a devastating effect on my health but we were desperate enough to consider even this possibility.

For a week, I kept right away from the kitchen, which was the only area where gas was used in summer time, and I stayed in our upstairs bedroom with all doors shut between me and the pilot light on the cooker. Each morning before he left home, Robin provided me with a Thermos flask of hot drink and some food to eat during the day. At the end of the week, I was very much better. We didn't have to think twice! Out went the cooker, together with all the gas pipes under the house, and we replaced it with a second-hand electric cooking stove. It made an enormous difference.

However, I soon discovered that I became ill again if I went into a house, a shop or a waiting room where there was gas – even if I didn't know it was there! In addition, it became clear that a whole host of other allergies had developed, and my doctor gave me non-stop prescriptions for antihistamines. Even on this medication, old allergies were very much worse. For instance, for several years prior to this, every spring time for about four months I felt dreadfully ill and my limbs were heavy and useless. The first time it happened, I was rushed to a London hospital for investigations, but they could find nothing wrong with me. After a few months, the symptoms simply subsided but, when they returned at the same time the following year – and the next, and the next – it was obvious that I had an allergy to some kind of spring-time pollen. Well, after being exposed to gas for a year, spring became an even worse nightmare.

In 1972, I hit rock bottom, both physically and mentally. The constant battle with my health had led to an anxiety state. At this point I discovered a new reality to my Christian faith and began to believe for my healing. I was determined to find out what had gone wrong with my body, and prayed as never before. Gradually, life became an adventure of discoveries and, one week after I had been prayed for by a Christian minister, I found I was completely healed of the gas allergy; it just never happened again, even though for a long time I was really scared of gas and expected the dreaded symptoms to return whenever I found myself in a house with a gas fire – such was the strength of my faith! But eventually I was convinced and one day we actually had gas re-piped to our house for central heating and two lovely open gas fires.

Yet other problems remained. At first, I could not understand why I should be healed of one problem but not the rest. I now believe it was because God had many things for me to learn, which would later be useful to pass on to others. For instance, I discovered how to regulate low blood sugar through diet, and how to control allergies with vitamins. I gave up coffee and cystitis disappeared!

I had an increasing conviction that nutrition held the key to all my remaining problems, yet I had never before given any thought whatsoever to the food I ate (except to enjoy it!) and I had certainly never seriously thought about what I should feed my children. I began to take stock of the situation, and to change our way of eating by discarding the attractively-packaged junk foods which I so often bought and beginning to learn instead how easy it was to use the healthy wholefoods which previously had been a mystery to me.

In 1985 I read about candidiasis – yeast infection – and *knew* it was the root of my problems. The information stated that, to bring candida under control, you needed a strict diet and a drug called Nystatin. I talked to my doctor and he ridiculed the whole idea and he certainly would not prescribe Nystatin, so the only thing I could do was to try the diet. For 18 months I kept to it rigidly. Even though nothing much happened, I knew I was on the right lines.

One day, I was amazed to hear from a friend that her doctor wanted to meet me. He had happened to say to her that he thought she might have yeast infection, to which she had replied that she was certain of it! He was surprised to find that she seemed to know more about the subject than he did, for it had only just begun to interest him, and he said that he would very much like to meet this friend who was apparently responsible for educating one of his patients! A meeting was set up and we had an interesting discussion, at the end of which I arranged to transfer to his practice. He was only too happy to prescribe Nystatin to see if it would help but, 18 months later, still on the diet as well as Nystatin, I was no better. At Christmas, I had contracted a virus and in the following April I was still sitting in a chair all day, trying to find enough energy to wash the breakfast dishes. It was in that April that I suggested to a few friends – all suspected 'yeasties' – that we should get together for the specific purpose of praying for an answer to our problems.

Within a week, the beginning of the answer was in my hands. Another friend lent me a copy of a magazine called *Here's Health*, and in it I read about a food supplement which was proving to be remarkably effective at destroying candida. It was caprylic acid, a fatty acid found in coconuts, which had apparently been known for many years to have anti-fungal properties. Students at the Institute for Optimum Nutrition in London were wanting volunteers suffering from candida (specifically vaginal thrush) to take part in a controlled trial with caprylic acid. I wrote off straight away but unfortunately the magazine was out of date and it was some time before I received a reply from the students to say I was too late to take part. In the meantime, I had managed to trace the suppliers of the caprylic acid supplement and I started on a course of it, still continuing with the diet and also taking other supplements called probiotics to reintroduce friendly bacteria – 'good guys' – into my intestines.

The immediate effect was discouraging because I felt ill and depressed and didn't know why this should be, but I was determined to persevere – and two months later I was a different woman! Not all the symptoms had yet disappeared, but I knew that my general health and stamina were better than I had ever known in my life before. In June 1988, I was able to drive to Cardiff in Wales from my home in Essex, not far from London, to collect our student daughter with all her belongings, drive around Wales with her for a couple of days, stop off to do some walking in the Brecon Beacons and then return home a long way round via Sussex in order to visit Robin who was spending three months at a Christian training centre. This amounted to not much less than a thousand miles of driving in just a few days – and I had never before had the stamina to drive more than 20 miles without being exhausted for the following week!

My doctor was very impressed with the improvement, and several friends, seeing the difference in me, started to ask my advice for their own health problems. I began to feel that I really needed to know rather more than I did about what I was doing. It's one thing to experiment with your own body, but quite another to take on the responsibility of advising other people. In any case, where do you start?

One day, I saw a notice in a health magazine announcing a two-year diploma course at the Institute for Optimum Nutrition in London – the establishment I had previously heard about in connection with the candida project. I was intrigued. As a grandmother now, could I possibly undertake such a training? And even if I could, would they accept me? It transpired that I could, they would and they did! I embarked on two years of very demanding study, working mostly at home but travelling to London for several weekends and seminars each term. Later, I returned for a third year of study but the initial two years provided the foundations of my new knowledge of nutrition. As I learned, more and more people contacted me for advice. I turned a bedroom into an office and started a card-index system. The telephone rang throughout each meal so we went out and bought an answerphone, and had another line installed so that family and friends could get through to us. Our lives were being taken over – but I loved every minute, enjoying the study and my new-found stamina to do all the work and still be able to cope with home, family and Christian involvements.

As I studied biochemistry and physiology, I came to realize the importance of nutrition to the efficient working of every single cell and system in the body. This was when I discovered that each one of us is different, and realized the importance of this concept of biochemical individuality. We were taught how to analyse and assess a person's nutritional status from very detailed questionnaires covering health history, current symptoms and daily eating habits. Therapeutic levels of vitamins and minerals were needed to make up deficiencies in nutritional status and to offset imbalances, and we were taught how to calculate these levels for each person so that a tailor-made programme of supplements could be formulated to meet specific needs.

I realized that this was the last piece of the puzzle in my understanding of how to beat candida. I had actually been taking vitamins and minerals for several years, working out my requirements as best I could from books such as *Let's Get Well* by Adelle Davis, but here was a way of calculating each person's requirements efficiently and effectively. And I realized that, through my own experience, a four-point plan had evolved for beating candida. First, it was necessary to starve the yeast by diet; second, it was essential to boost the immune system with a tailor-made programme of vitamins and minerals; third, antifungal supplements were necessary to actually destroy the yeast; and, fourth, probiotic supplements were needed to re-establish a healthy colony of friendly bacteria.

I steered other people on to this four-point plan and found increasingly that their health improved. They really began to get well. One man aged 42, suffering from diagnosed ME, had been unable to work for the past two years and could walk only 100 yards, leaning on a stick. After five months on the four-point plan, he went back to work part-time and soon was able to cope with full-time employment. A young friend who had been suffering from weakness and fatigue for seven years, since having glandular fever, soon felt such a return of energy that one Saturday she cycled 15 miles with her husband and went to a barn dance in the evening. It was getting pretty exciting!

Others were taking considerably longer to improve and I tried to discover what might be holding them back. In the process, I learned about die-off reaction or, to use its proper name, *Herxheimer* reaction. I have already said that live candida releases 79 identified chemical toxins; I now have to tell you that dead candida releases even more! The more candida you destroy, the worse you are likely to feel as all these extra toxins invade your bloodstream, leading to a worsening of all your symptoms including aches and pains, a muzzy head and depression. I found that people would possibly discontinue the anti-candida diet because they felt ill on it, or else thought they were allergic to caprylic acid when they started taking antifungals. These people needed to have die-off explained to them so that they saw these unpleasant symptoms as an encouragement, a sign that candida in their bodies was being brought under control rather than getting worse, as they had thought. They also needed to be told ways of alleviating the symptoms of die-off reaction.

I soon began to discover other reasons why some people made slow progress, and I shall say more about these in Chapter 4, but such problems are not always present, by any means. Time and again I see people improve beyond recognition over the course of a few months, simply by following the four-point plan.

My own battle with candida, fought hard and long, eventually led me to become a qualified Nutrition Consultant, gaining my diploma from the Institute for Optimum Nutrition in 1990 with Distinction. I learned, and have since experienced many times over, how nutritional advice can help people to overcome an enormous number of health problems. For instance, I carried out a research project into eating disorders as part of my training, having become aware of the tragic suffering which accompanies such disorders as anorexia and bulimia nervosa, and I was amazed at what could be achieved by using a complex of amino acids.

I have frequently seen stubbornly high blood pressure respond to simple changes in diet and a few food supplements; the miseries of premenstrual syndrome disappear; hyperactive children become a joy to live with; and painful conditions like arthritis and neuritis brought under control. Eczema and psoriasis clear, allergic reactions to cats and dogs no longer occur, irritable bowel syndrome becomes a thing of the past, depression and anxiety are forgotten – I have even seen tremendous improvements in schizophrenia when a co-operative consultant has allowed me access to a hospitalized patient.

Each day brings the reward of hearing that clients are experiencing increasing health and happiness. One young woman, suffering from extreme overweight, had been told by a hospital specialist that her condition was hereditary and nothing could be done to help her. He added that they would try to 'keep her going until she was 40'. As she was then 33, she was living under a seven-year death-sentence. Nobody had considered that her problem might be due to food allergy, fluid retention – and candida! Just six weeks into the four-point plan, she had lost two stones in weight, and after six months she had lost six stones!

In the first edition of this book, I wrote that I had seen all this and more, and yet at that time I had been qualified and in practice for little more than a year. I soon became so busy that my husband, Robin, left teaching in order to take over the administration of my growing practice. It is now nine years since I qualified and I have seen an enormous number of people, suffering from a wide variety of health problems, come through to a state of fully-restored health through achieving optimum nutrition and, where necessary, following the anti-candida four-point plan.

I soon discovered that, because I could carry out a symptoms' analysis from detailed questionnaires, it was possible to work from our home in the South-East of England and help people by post in the far north of Scotland and, later, in Europe, Scandinavia, the Far East, the Middle East, Australasia and the USA! None of this would have been possible if I had not first experienced the many years of suffering due to candida, and found a way to beat it. Eleven years on and into my sixties, I have the health and stamina to cope with an enormous workload which includes consultations, writing and lecturing, both in the UK and abroad. I rejoice in the health which for so long eluded me and, because it happened for me, I have the confidence to believe that it can happen for others, also.

By far the largest proportion of people who contact me have candida and many of these have ME. Although trained to help with a wide assortment of health problems, I find myself increasingly working with people who are suffering just as I once did. I work closely with the chief Consultant Neurologist who specialises in ME and, in the vast majority of cases, the results achieved by nutritional therapy are most encouraging.

For many people, just hearing an explanation of what is probably causing their problems brings a ray of hope after months or even years of fruitless medical investigations. The first thing they need to do is to check out their candida score at the back of this book. If there is the slightest possibility that they might have yeast infection, they then need to be pointed towards the anti-candida four-point plan which changed my life. Let's have a look at it in a little more detail.

Chapter 3

The Four-point Plan

The strategy which I have found to be effective for bringing Candida albicans under control takes the form of a four-point plan:

1) A strict anti-yeast diet to starve the candida.
2) An individually tailor-made supplement programme providing vitamins and minerals to boost the immune system.
3) Natural antifungal supplements to kill the candida.
4) Friendly bacteria to help restore a healthy balance of microbes in the intestines.

Many times people say to me, 'I've been on an anti-candida diet and it hasn't helped at all,' or, 'I've taken lots of vitamins but it's made no difference,' or even, 'I've tried caprylic acid supplements and they just made me worse – I think I must have been allergic to them' – this last situation usually being die-off reaction for which the sufferer has not been prepared.

What I have found over and over again is that all four points of this plan need to be followed; if one of them is left out – no matter which one – it really doesn't work. Each of the four points is of equal importance, but on its own is unlikely to have an effect – certainly no lasting effect. Let's look at the four points one at a time.

1. The Anti-candida Diet

The purpose of the diet is to starve candida to death! Sugar is known to activate yeast, and it will do it just as well in your colon as in a mixing bowl. This means that all types of sugar – whether sucrose (white table sugar), raw cane sugar, demerara, glucose, fructose, dextrose, honey or even lactose (the natural sugar in milk) – have to be totally avoided. Some foods quickly turn to glucose in the blood, especially refined grains like white flour, white rice and cornflour (cornstarch), and these are just as dangerous as actual sugar. The total avoidance of all forms of sugar is one of the biggest hurdles to climb, but if you are determined to get well, you will soon decide that giving up sweet things is really not such a sacrifice when you consider the rewards it will bring. I usually find that, after a month or so on the diet, most people are already well on the way to losing their 'sweet tooth' and, with it, their craving for those foods which feed the candida.

One of the hardest things for people to understand is that, if you are trying to beat candida, fruit is no good for you. We are so accustomed to thinking of fruit as the most healthy food available (which of course it is, if you haven't got yeast infection) that we cannot cope with the idea of a fruitless diet. The fructose it contains is as good as a spoonful of treacle if you happen to be a candida spore. Sugar is sugar! To some people, the idea of not having fruit juice comes even harder. 'But it's natural and unsweetened!' Drinking a glass of orange juice is like drinking a glass of straight sugar solution, and your candida will love it! Some practitioners and authors say that you need only exclude fruit for a short time, varying from three weeks to three months. In my experience, if you put fruit back into your diet before you are completely well, it will slow down or even completely block your recovery, so I take a very firm line on this. Maybe this is different from other advice you've been given, but then maybe that is why you still need to look for help!

In Chapter 4, you will find guidelines for the anti-candida diet. You will see that there are other things to be avoided, besides sugar. Foods containing yeast (for instance, yeasted bread, yeast spreads and gravy mixes) have to go, as does anything fermented (vinegar and alcohol), anything containing mould (cheese and cured or smoked fish and meat) and stimulants (tea, coffee, chocolate, cola drinks). One effect of a stimulant is to provoke the adrenal glands to trigger the release of the body's sugar stores into the bloodstream, in just the same way as stress, and this sugar will feed candida as effectively as sugar which has just been eaten!

A tremendous number of people are amazed at how much better they feel once they have given up tea and coffee. We look upon these drinks as a harmless part of our civilized culture, but in fact tea, coffee, chocolate and cola drinks each contain several addictive stimulants which cause all sorts of problems from migraine to anxiety, depression, insomnia and palpitations. Even beverages which have had their caffeine removed still contain other stimulating substances – theophylline, theobromine, tannin – and they are just as addictive as caffeine. You need to find alternative drinks which you enjoy and then just make up your mind to stop drinking tea and coffee. If you try to wean yourself off them gradually, almost certainly it will not work! Choose a weekend, perhaps, when there is not much to do, because you will quite probably have a headache. This is because you will be experiencing withdrawal symptoms from all those stimulant drugs in your favourite drinks. Take a painkiller, if necessary, to help you through it, and in a couple of days you will start to feel better than you have for a long time – but make sure you don't take one of the common painkillers which contain caffeine. Many do, and obviously this would defeat the object of the exercise.

Apart from the anti-candida diet guidelines in Chapter 6, please read carefully the guidelines in Chapter 7 which give you some other good advice on healthy eating. The right oils and margarines, for instance, make so much difference to our health and, in order to get rid of the candida overgrowth, you need to build up your body in every way possible. Besides this, once you have learned these new eating habits, you will be laying an excellent foundation for your future health.

Starting on the anti-candida diet and keeping to it is not helped by the fact that candidiasis actually produces a craving for things like sugar, fruit, alcohol, bread, cheese and chocolate. The yeast in your body seems to demand what *it* needs in order to survive and to thrive! These demands bypass the good intentions of your mind, and sometimes you find yourself guiltily giving in to an uncontrollable binge because the craving is so powerful. It might also be due to the fact that you have low blood sugar, which will not in fact improve by putting more sugar into your body! That just makes the situation worse and is another instance when your body really doesn't know what's best for it. I'll explain more about low blood sugar later on.

Another situation which triggers cravings is food allergy. Allergy often equals addiction. If you are unknowingly addicted to something, possibly tea or coffee, chocolate, alcohol, or even wheat or potatoes – whatever it might be – you begin to get withdrawal symptoms when some time has elapsed since you last ate or drank it. Almost certainly, you will not recognize these symptoms for what they are; you just feel a bit 'low', or tired, or have a headache. Because you don't feel too well, you turn to the very thing which you know will make you feel better – for a while, at any rate; a cup of tea, a glass of wine, a bar of chocolate, a bread roll, some potato crisps. Your body is telling you what it thinks it needs – and once again you are feeding your addiction. This is a pretty good indication that you are in fact allergic to the very substance which you have been eating or drinking several times each day.

If you have a real problem with craving, you may need specific help to overcome it so that you can cope with the demands of the anti-candida diet. If you consult a nutritionist who decides that you have symptoms associated with low blood sugar, the recommendations in your tailor-made supplement programme will take account of it. If you find you have an uncontrollable craving for sweet things or for alcohol, you could try an amino acid called L-Glutamine, available in supplement form, which will help to control the craving until you have lost your sweet tooth and find that keeping to the diet is no longer a problem.

Later, I shall talk about how and when you can experiment with relaxing the diet. At this stage, I want not only to stress the importance of this particular diet but also to encourage you to have the right attitude towards it. If you look upon this as a time of misery and of being deprived of the things you most enjoy, you will have great difficulty in overcoming candida, and probably find some excuse for not embarking on the four-point plan. Such clients are sometimes quite aggressive to me, saying that this regime is 'too extreme and radical'. What they really mean is that they don't intend to give up drinking coffee!

If, on the other hand, you are determined to get well by doing everything you can to help yourself, you will find that the diet is not so bad after all and you will soon discover that you really quite enjoy all the foods which are allowed. Not everything which has to be avoided in the diet will need to be excluded for ever, once candida is under control, but a substance like sugar will only encourage the yeast to thrive again, as well as causing other problems, so why not learn to enjoy life without it? It really can be done!

2. Personal Supplement Programme

Just as important as the diet is the need to boost the efficiency of your immune system by taking food supplements – vitamins, minerals, essential fatty acids and possibly amino acids – at levels which have been calculated to meet your own personal optimum daily requirement. You will find help for doing this in *The Optimum Nutrition Bible* by Patrick Holford, or you might prefer to consult a qualified nutritionist to calculate your requirements and formulate your tailor-made programme of supplements. Learning how to do this was an important part of my training at the Institute for Optimum Nutrition in London. The recommendations are based on therapeutic levels of specific nutrients, which are obviously well within the safety margins for toxicity. My experience is that if these initial levels are maintained for three months, a review of the situation after that time will usually show that many of the symptoms have disappeared, which means that levels of nutrients may be reduced accordingly. Eventually, maintenance levels will be all that is needed to keep the immune system boosted and the body functioning efficiently, but this will usually take longer than three months to achieve so the situation needs to be monitored at regular intervals.

The questionnaire on which I base my recommendations was devised by the Institute for Optimum Nutrition, although it has been adapted to include a score for candida symptoms and has a few refinements for ease of working. The completed questionnaire reveals all sorts of things to the trained eye. For instance, various symptoms are associated with a deficiency of a particular vitamin or mineral; to choose a simple example, white marks on the fingernails indicate a lack of zinc, an important mineral which is needed by an enormous number of cells and functions in the body. The questionnaire also highlights symptoms associated with low blood sugar, low or high histamine status, high cardiovascular (heart) risk, hormone imbalance, allergy and stress potential, thyroid efficiency and pollution risks. All these situations may be helped by taking the right level of certain vitamins, minerals and essential fatty acids, at the same time as making appropriate changes in diet. For example, if you have a high risk of aluminium toxicity (from taking lots of indigestion tablets and cooking in aluminium pans, for instance), the level of aluminium being taken up by your body may actually be reduced by taking the right amounts of vitamins C and B_6 together with the minerals calcium, magnesium and zinc. Pectin and alginic acid (from seaweed) also help, as do foods which contain sulphur, like eggs and onions. (Other ways in which we absorb aluminium are from drinking water, toothpaste, aspirin and most types of antiperspirant.)

If I am concerned about the possibility of high levels of toxic metals from pollution, I sometimes suggest a hair mineral analysis. The most recent growth of hair is a pretty good indicator of levels of minerals in the body, and will help to show if you are deficient in essential minerals or have too much of a toxic metal like mercury, lead or aluminium. Heavy metal toxicity can cause all sorts of problems from hyperactivity and learning difficulties in children to unexplained neuralgia or neuritis in an adult. It has been acknowledged by the British Medical Association that high levels of aluminium are often associated with Alzheimer's disease, a form of senility. At the very least, too much of any heavy metal in your body will put a load on your immune system and so weaken it in its fight against candida. The results of the hair mineral analysis are taken into account when calculating or adjusting your requirements for specific vitamins and minerals.

Incidentally, if high levels of mercury are indicated because you have a large number of amalgam fillings in your teeth, I do not in fact recommend having the fillings replaced too soon because the large amount of mercury vapour released in the process puts a tremendous load on the immune system and will sometimes cause a severe flare-up of candida problems, even when the dentist has been well-trained in preventative measures to be taken during the process. A change-over to less toxic fillings is something which can be considered when your nutritional status has been built up and the immune system has begun to get stronger. However, for future fillings you should ask to have porcelain or whatever alternative substance your dentist recommends.

As I have said, discovering how to calculate optimum levels of nutrients was, for me, like finding the missing piece of a jigsaw puzzle. I cannot stress too strongly that, unless the immune system is boosted by being given the right levels of the right kind of 'fuel' to repair the machinery and help it to run efficiently, you might just as well not bother with the rest of the four-point plan.

Neither can I stress too strongly that each person's requirements are unique to them and to their present situation. I analyse several questionnaires each day, and I am constantly struck by the fact that, although several clients might be suffering from an overgrowth of candida, their individual needs for vitamins and minerals are completely different. When I was trying to work out my own requirements, I dipped into many different books on nutrition to find out which supplements I needed and how much I should take of each one. It was a long and arduous task, and I now know that my efforts were ignorant of such factors as pollution levels and histamine status, so I feel certain that I would have made a speedier recovery had I known all the factors involved and been able to take them into account in my original attempt to formulate a supplement programme for myself.

Clients often say to me that they have taken vitamins for years, to which my reply is that they cannot have been doing them very much good, otherwise there would be no need for this present consultation! When I look at the packet they have brought to show me, I have to tell them that they have really been wasting their money because the levels of nutrients contained in the product are far below the client's actual requirements. Worse still, very often the supplements they have been taking contain yeast, which has been encouraging candida to thrive rather than boosting the client's immune system to fight it. With vitamins and minerals, it is essential to know what you are doing and get your programme right.

My personal philosophy is that, even when we are completely well, we can only benefit from a few pence spent each day on food supplements to help make up for the many deficiencies in adulterated and depleted food so that our bodies can then cope with the many varied effects of pollution. I really believe that we cannot expect to have automatic good health any longer, because we have messed up our food and our environment to such an extent that our immune system is in constant danger of breaking down under the load. However, I also believe that it is still possible to experience one hundred per cent health if we are prepared to do something about it by eating as healthily as possible and by taking supplements to make up for the remaining deficiencies. Not only will this help to protect our bodies against pollution but it will also give them a greater chance of being able to avoid future yeast problems and of being able to stand firm against attempted attacks by other disease-causing micro-organisms.

Once you are well, a good once-daily multivitamin and mineral complex will probably suffice, although you still need to take into account any special situations. For instance, if you have amalgam fillings, they will constantly release mercury vapour so your body needs help to off-load it by taking good levels of vitamin C, zinc and selenium. Another case for special consideration is a woman who has reached menopause, because she needs the right levels of magnesium, calcium (in a form which is well-absorbed, such as citrate or succinate) and vitamin D in order to guard against the onset of osteoporosis.

When you do eventually reach the stage of needing just a maintenance programme, your nutritionist will be able to advise you on supplements which are best suited to your ongoing needs. Meanwhile, let the therapeutic levels in your recommended programme help you to achieve your optimum nutritional status.

It needs to be said that there are two situations which often prevent even the right levels of supplements from producing this improvement. The first is that the digestive system might not be working efficiently, which means that the body is not absorbing adequate nutrients, and the second situation is that smoking cigarettes will literally block the absorption of some nutrients and destroy others. Digestion and absorption can be helped by your nutritionist who will suggest that you include some digestive enzymes in your programme; the second situation really requires that you make a decision to stop smoking – or at least to cut down drastically in the first place to fewer than five cigarettes per day. If you want to be well, if you want to overcome candida, it is up to you to stop smoking. That may sound hard but I'm afraid it's simply the fact of the matter. And you will be so glad that you did!

So now we have covered the first two points of the four-point plan: the anti-candida diet and the tailor-made supplement programme. I recommend that my clients should follow these two points of the plan for at least a month before progressing to points 3 and 4. There are several reasons for this.

First, it can take a while to get used to the diet. For some people, it is an incredibly radical change to their eating habits, and they might not be able to sort it all out straight away. Second, the vitamins and minerals will have their own work to do before adding extra supplements. They will start to correct deficiencies and imbalances, and in so doing they will help to put the immune system in better fighting shape than it has probably been for a very long time. But the main reason I want them to wait for a month is because I need to see what is going to happen. Two things are possible. Once the first week is over (when there is often a headache due to coming off tea and coffee), clients will quite often start to feel better than they have for years. This is not surprising, because they are eating a good healthy diet which contains no sugar or other junk foods, and they are also taking plenty of vitamins and minerals. If they feel pretty good at the end of the month, there is no problem at all in progressing to points 3 and 4.

However, rather more often, clients report that they feel worse as the month goes on. They might think they have influenza, and yet there is no high temperature. They might feel nauseous or have diarrhoea, or they might be very depressed. Almost without exception, they tell me that they feel even more fatigued than before, that their arms and legs are aching, and that their heads feel 'muzzy' so that they cannot think or remember clearly. Old symptoms like eczema, sinusitis or vaginal thrush flare up badly, and the client rings me up to say, 'I'm so disappointed; I just feel worse. I'm afraid your programme isn't working for me.'

To which I reply, 'Oh, yes it is!' In fact, nothing could be more certain! What they are experiencing is Herxheimer reaction, or 'die-off'. This does not mean, however, that the client is dying off! It means that candida is already being starved to death by the diet and further pushed back by an immune system which is beginning to grow stronger. Since dead yeast releases a great many extra toxins, it is not surprising that you don't feel well until the body has been able to off-load them. Not only is your bloodstream full of toxic substances, but each area of your body which has been colonized by candida is now having to deal with toxins being released by dead candida in those very areas, so for a while the inflammation in joints or skin or sinuses or other tissues is worse than it was before.

Taking antifungal supplements a little later on can have the same effect, but at that stage you are able to control the severity of 'die-off' by adjusting the level of antifungals which you take in a day. However, when die-off occurs simply as a result of starting the diet and taking some vitamins, you need to do something to alleviate the symptoms. Make sure that you drink plenty of water, and you can also take vitamin C to what is known as 'bowel tolerance levels' – in other words, until it causes you to have a loose bowel motion. When the body is full of toxins (and also when it is fighting an infection or an allergy), its tissues will soak up vitamin C like a sponge, so you can sometimes take very large amounts before it causes a loose stool. The next day you will usually find that it takes a little less, and so on. It is also important to support the liver in its detoxification work, and this is discussed in more detail later on.

Obviously, if die-off is unpleasant, you do not want to add to the symptoms by killing off even more yeast in your body, so it is best to wait until the symptoms have improved before taking antifungal supplements. As soon as you feel on a reasonably 'even keel', you can move on to this next stage of the four-point plan, but I hope you can see why it is that I advise you to wait at least a month before you do.

In my practice, my clients know that they can keep in close telephone contact with me so that they can check out what is happening to them. This means that, together, we can make the decision about when is the right time to move on to points 3 and 4 of the four-point plan. I also prepare them in advance to understand about die-off reaction by providing an audiotape which I have recorded, and this helps them to welcome the symptoms with the knowledge that candida is now being destroyed. Psychologically, this is far more helpful than being left to think that the diet or the vitamins are making them become more ill.

3. Antifungal Supplements

The products which I recommend in my practice most frequently are the same ones which helped me so much, and which I have now seen work effectively in countless other lives.

There are in fact different types of antifungals, but I normally recommend starting with caprylic acid, a fatty acid found in coconuts. It was known in the 1930s that coconuts had antifungal properties but, until the last few years, they had not been fully studied. Now caprylic acid is available as a well-researched, natural antifungal substance. I use calcium magnesium caprylate, which is the most useful way of taking caprylic acid because it ensures that it will reach the large intestine, the root area of all other problems of candida overgrowth. It is possible to find capsules containing sodium caprylate but, since sodium is absorbed from the small intestine, the caprylic acid would never reach the colon. Of course, other practitioners often recommend other methods of using these products, but this is an approach which makes good sense, and I have seen it be effective many thousands of times.

Calcium magnesium caprylate may be bought in three strengths, with capsules containing 250 mg, 400 mg and 680 mg. I use the 250 mg strength with children, but also with some adults who experience very severe die-off effects. More often, I start by recommending the 400 mg capsules, taking just one daily with a meal. In this way, my clients will normally avoid having strong die-off symptoms but, if they do, they may either persevere for a day or two to see if the situation will improve or else they let me know and I will take them off caprylic acid for a time and take more steps to improve the liver's detoxification processes, as I shall discuss in a moment.

However, if taking a 400 mg capsule each day has not led to die-off reaction after five days, clients may then increase to two capsules daily, one with breakfast and one with their evening meal, and continue for another five days. Very gradually, in this way, they increase the level until eventually they are on six capsules every day, taking two with each meal. If, at any stage along the way, die-off reaction becomes too unpleasant, the level should certainly not be increased and may even be decreased until the symptoms subside, which will indicate that the body has eliminated the current load of toxins released by dead candida.

There is only one way in which you can be certain that the symptoms you are experiencing are caused by die-off toxins rather than a flare-up of candida activity, and that is to be equally certain that you are doing absolutely everything in your power to destroy candida. In other words, if you are keeping strictly to the diet without cheating and taking all the supplements needed to boost your immune system, it is simply not possible for candidiasis to become worse, so the symptoms you are experiencing *must* be due to die-off! However, if you start feeling worse and have been cheating on your diet, there is no way of telling whether you are in fact experiencing a certain amount of die-off reaction or whether a new flare-up of candida activity is responsible for your symptoms. It is virtually impossible to sort out what is happening, so it is really best to stick strictly to the diet so that you can be absolutely certain that an increase of symptoms means die-off reaction!

Once my clients have reached the point of taking six capsules of the 400 mg capsule each day *without experiencing die-off symptoms*, quite often I suggest that they move on to the 680 mg capsules, starting with three capsules daily and once more increasing gradually to six capsules daily, taking two with each meal. Caprylic acid is an excellent antifungal substance for dealing with candida in the intestines. To some extent it is also absorbed into other tissues of the body but, being a long-chain fatty acid, it has some difficulty in penetrating fatty cell wall membranes. On the other hand, there are antifungal plant oils which have a short-chain fatty acid structure, and these are able to penetrate outlying tissues in the body (muscles, joints, skin, sinuses, etc.) far more easily. The oils of cloves, artemisia and oregano are often very helpful once gastrointestinal symptoms have improved but other symptoms remain. As with caprylic acid, they should be increased cautiously from one to two capsules per day, but they are so well absorbed that they do not need to be increased above two daily. Whether or not a client transfers to 680 mg of caprylic acid or to the herbal oils depends on whether or not caprylic acid still seems to be having an effect – in other words, whether there was a temporary increase of die-off symptoms when making the last jump with 400 mg capsules from five to six daily. If it is still doing some work, stay with caprylic acid for a longer period of time; if not, change to the other approach.

When a client has been symptom-free for a few weeks without having any die-off reaction, and provided this improvement is confirmed by a candida score which is close to zero (allowing for an ongoing score for predisposing factors, of course), we can then consider undertaking a gentle experiment with relaxing the anti-candida diet for one month – in sensible ways, for which I provide guidelines.

Antifungal supplements should be continued during this stage, in case one or other of the newly-restored foods still manages to cause a flare-up of symptoms by slightly reactivating some candida. If this should happen, the diet-relax experiment should be stopped and the antifungals will quickly bring the situation under control once more. The programme then needs to be resumed for a little longer, possibly a month or two, before trying the experiment again.

If all goes well during the one month's experiment, this is an encouraging sign that candida overgrowths are now fairly well under control and both antifungal and probiotic supplements (point 4 of the four-point plan) may be stopped. However, it is important to stay on maintenance levels of vitamins and minerals to keep your immune system strong and, if you were to stay on a relaxed diet at this early stage, I'm afraid you would re-encourage your candida to be active and quite soon be back where you started. Later, I shall explain the way ahead with the diet in more detail (see pages 42–5).

Sometimes a client will do very well for a while but then seem to reach a 'plateau' – a level at which he or she is certainly feeling better than they were to start with, but not improving to a point of total victory. This might be an indication that yeasts other than Candida albicans have gained a foothold, or that intestinal parasites are complicating the situation, so supplements are needed which have a more broad-spectrum effect than caprylic acid. Such a situation might be suspected when the illness originated in a hot climate where there was something to be desired in terms of the water supply and environmental hygiene. Although the accuracy and usefulness of tests for candida are debatable, a diagnostic stool test can be extremely helpful in deciding which herbal or nutritional products are likely to be most effective when it comes to specific forms of bacteria or parasites.

Garlic has undoubted broad-spectrum properties, and many people take great quantities of it in an effort to bring their bad guys under control. However, having such effective broad-spectrum effects means that it also kills off the good guys! One use of garlic capsules which I discovered for myself was in dealing with the soreness and pain caused by candida in my mouth. Frequently, it would flare up along my gums and affect the nerves of my teeth. The pain was excruciating! The only thing which helped was to cut open a garlic capsule and rub the oil on my gums. For years I went to bed every night smelling strongly of garlic. Fortunately, I had a long-suffering husband! Even so, although the garlic oil brought great relief, the condition never totally cleared and I realized later that, besides killing candida, garlic was also destroying the friendly bacteria in my mouth. Eventually I discovered that propolis tincture did a far better job. Propolis is made by bees and has effective antifungal, antibacterial and anti-parasitic properties, as well as being slightly anaesthetic and therefore soothing, but it does not disturb the good guys!

Nutritional therapy is a bit like taking layers off an onion. You see how far you can get with one approach and, if necessary, move on to another. That is how it is with the different types of natural antifungal products now available to us.

4. Beneficial Bacteria

The fourth part of the four-point plan is to include supplements which will reintroduce beneficial bacteria to the intestines so that a healthy colony of good guys is quickly re-established. These helpful supplements are called probiotics.

One of the friendly bacteria is Lactobacillus acidophilus, commonly found in yoghurt so, unless you have an intolerance to dairy foods, it is good to eat plenty of low-fat, natural yoghurt. However, not very much yoghurt will actually reach the colon which is where you need to re-establish a healthy colony of friendly bacteria. For this reason, it is good to use a capsule containing freeze-dried Lactobacillus acidophilus together with Lactobacillus bifidobacteria, because these two good guys enhance each other's effectiveness. I recommend a capsule containing over four billion live organisms, taking one twice daily. There is no need to increase or decrease it as you do with antifungals; you simply take one with breakfast and one with supper all the time you are taking any type of antifungal supplements. (Some product labels state that it should be taken before meals and others after, depending on the process of production, level of stability, etc., so read the instructions carefully for maximum benefit. These products are always best kept in a refrigerator.)

So there you have it, the anti-candida four-point plan, as I discovered and experienced it for myself and have since found to be effective many times over. Given time, and with determination and perseverance, I believe it is impossible for it *not* to bring candida under control. However, there may be other situations which are holding back your recovery and which therefore need to be found and dealt with, and this requires a certain amount of detective work.

Chapter 4

Possible Problems Holding Back Your Recovery

Environmental Allergies

It might be that you are reacting to something in the environment because of your weakened immune system. I have already described the horrendous effects I experienced from North Sea gas when it was first piped into houses in England. Some people are being made ill by all sorts of other chemical smells, without realizing it. I use a simple questionnaire to help try to pinpoint any of these possible factors.

House plants are a problem because the soil in the pot contains mould spores which become airborne, and a yeast-sensitive person will breathe them in and react to them. Many people feel as sentimental about their house plants as they do about their pets, and strongly resist my advice to foster them out or give them away, yet doing so can make an enormous difference to their symptoms and to the speed of their overall recovery.

In fact, mould anywhere in the house – under sinks, in cellars or bathrooms, around double-glazed windows – can cause a very bad reaction in a 'yeasty' person and also hold back their recovery by placing an ongoing load on the immune system. Quite a few people take a giant step forward when the mould has been dealt with and removed from their environment. Damp places in the house need priority attention, so watch out for mottled patches on wallpaper or musty smells in cupboards – tell-tale signs of damp and mould. Autumn walks among rotting leaves had a dreadful effect on me, and I always anticipate an influx of telephone calls when leaves are on the ground and the weather is dank and misty. You can almost smell mushrooms growing! I once visited a very musty-smelling castle in Northumberland, in the North of England, and the rest of my holiday was a total write-off!

Severe Die-off Reaction

Sometimes, people find it extremely difficult to increase (or even to start taking) their antifungal supplements. They experience so much die-off reaction that they really cannot cope with it. There are several possible explanations.

Constipation

Many of the toxins produced by dead candida will find their way into the faeces so, if you are constipated, the toxins will be reabsorbed into your bloodstream through your colon wall. This will happen all the more readily if you have a porous intestinal wall, known as a 'leaky gut'. Constipation must be avoided at all costs, and yet it is a very common problem.

For a long time, your body has been used to working with an incorrect balance of microbes in your intestines; now that the situation is being corrected, it leads to a disruption. Sometimes this disruption causes a phase of diarrhoea, sometimes constipation. At least diarrhoea gets rid of the toxins!

The anti-candida diet is based on natural wholefoods which are high in fibre, so don't take added bran (which acts like steel wool on your intestinal lining, causing excess mucus to be produced in an attempt to protect itself). However, linseeds or psyllium husks might be a useful addition in helping to avoid constipation. You should also drink plenty of water and take vitamin C to bowel tolerance levels – till you experience a loose motion, which tells you that you have taken enough vitamin C for that day.

A Toxic Liver

Long-term medication, or a history of drug or alcohol abuse, will have left toxic residues in the liver so that the arrival on the scene of lots more toxins from dead candida is just too much for the liver to cope with. Fortunately, nutritional steps can be taken to help detoxify the liver, and this alone will sometimes make a tremendous difference to symptoms. Then, after a few weeks, it is possible to start taking antifungals again – and this time, hopefully, the body will be able to cope with the extra toxins being released.

First steps to take to help detoxify the liver include a herbal supplement containing silymarin, or milk thistle, and 'coffee' made from dandelion root, roasted or unroasted, which stimulates the production of bile, the substance which carries toxins out of the liver. You should not buy dandelion coffee in a jar because it probably contains lactose. To make it yourself using the root pieces (available in packets from good health-food stores), look up the recipe in the Drinks section (*see page 154*).

If these simple steps are not sufficient, other nutritional steps are needed. Detoxification in the liver takes place in two stages, known as Phase I and Phase II. Phase I takes toxins from the blood and turns them into even more toxic substances in order to trigger Phase II into action, which then neutralizes the toxins, making them ready to be off-loaded. However, long-term ill-health with its attendant long-term medication has frequently led to a situation where Phase II is exhausted, so there is a build-up of toxins as they enter Phase I but no way for them to be neutralized and eliminated. In this situation, it can become increasingly difficult to take antifungal supplements because, as more and more candida is destroyed, it leads to an increasing build-up of toxins which are absorbed back into the body. Fortunately, specific nutrients are known to stimulate Phase II and so help to break the vicious cycle, and a laboratory test is available (in the USA, but also through nutritionists in the UK and elsewhere) to help confirm the situation, but I strongly advise you to enlist the help of a qualified nutritionist if you suspect that this might be relevant in your own situation.

Allergy to Die-off Toxins

Another possible explanation for severe die-off reaction is that, in a person who tends to suffer from allergies, their immune system might be reacting to the toxins produced by dead candida. This means that the die-off effect is twice as bad as it would otherwise be. A clue to this possibility is when part of the die-off effect includes mental or emotional problems – depression, anxiety, panic, irritability, mood swings – because this is how the 'allergic' reaction frequently shows itself. These people are able to cope better with the effect of antifungal supplements if they are also taking specific food supplements to reduce their allergic potential. They certainly played an important part in my own recovery when I found that by far the worst symptoms of die-off – worse than all the aches and pains, unpleasant as they were – were morbid depression and acute anxiety. Discovering the allergy factor made all the difference in enabling me to persevere with taking antifungals.

Poor Digestion and Absorption

With some people, slow progress is simply a question of faulty digestion and absorption so that they do not receive the benefit of their immune-boosting supplements. This needs help from digestive enzymes and it is also possible that steps need to be taken to encourage the production of hydrochloric acid in the stomach. Many people suffer from digestive symptoms which they put down to having too much acid. In fact, it is impossible to tell from your symptoms whether you have too much or too little acid, because the symptoms of each condition are the same! You can see from this that constantly sucking antacid tablets might well be having an entirely counter-productive effect. There is a simple way of finding out whether you have insufficient stomach acid – eat some beetroot and then watch the colour of your urine. Hydrochloric acid is needed to break down the colouring in the beetroot so, if your urine has a distinct red colour, you can be certain that you are low in stomach acid – and should not be taking antacid preparations for your indigestion.

Bacteria or Parasites

If you have a history of illness contracted overseas, it is possible that you might be harbouring a parasite as well as an overgrowth of candida, or there might be an overgrowth of bacteria. In these situations, a diagnostic laboratory test can be extremely useful. Great Smokies Laboratory in North Carolina, USA, offers a diagnostic package (available through nutritionists, see below) which includes a Comprehensive Digestive Stool Analysis plus Parasitology and also a urine test to show the level of intestinal permeability, indicating whether (or to what extent) a leaky gut is encouraging food intolerance and also allowing toxins and bacteria to invade the bloodstream. Once you know what you're up against, a great deal can be done, nutritionally, to improve matters.

Food Allergy

Food sensitivity or intolerance (most frequently referred to as 'allergy') is often a major factor in candida problems. In the same way as an overloaded immune system cannot cope efficiently with an invading bacteria or virus, neither can it cope with certain foods. However, I have now seen that there are very few of these offending substances which we will need to avoid for the rest of our lives, if only we take steps to strengthen the immune system, heal the intestinal wall and boost the production of digestive enzymes, but, in the first place it is necessary to discover the offending substances and avoid them so that a degree of load is removed from the immune system, allowing it more resources with which to fight candida.

The first foods to suspect are those which appear most frequently in the three-day food diary which I ask my clients to keep. This is because we frequently become addicted to the very foods which our immune systems have difficulty tolerating. To check out a suspect food, I tell my clients how to carry out a pulse test. You need to avoid the food for a minimum of five days (which allows time for your immune system to forget how to tolerate it), then find a time when you can sit still for just over an hour, taking with you some of the food to be tested. After five minutes of sitting still, you take your resting pulse rate and write it down. You then eat the food, continuing to sit still, and take your pulse again after 10 minutes, again after 30 minutes, and again at the end of an hour. Each time, take your pulse for a full minute and write it down. An intolerance or sensitivity to a food is very often shown by a rise (or sometimes a fall) in pulse rate. Sometimes the initial reaction is a rise followed later by a fall. There might also be some clear manifestation in other ways over the next 24 hours because, after a break of five days, the immune system might well react to it more strongly than before, giving rise to obvious symptoms.

If a suspect food is a member of a common food family, the whole family should be avoided simultaneously so that reactions are not masked. (For example, the gluten family includes wheat, oats, rye and barley; the nightshade family includes potatoes, tomatoes, peppers and aubergines or eggplants; and the dairy family includes yoghurt, cottage cheese and butter.) Each food within the family is then tested individually at 48-hour intervals. This doesn't mean that you will necessarily react to all the foods in a certain family – but, on the other hand, you might, and you really need to know.

If the overall change in pulse rate (from highest to lowest or the other way round) is 10 beats or more per minute, either up or down, or if there are unpleasant symptoms, it is important to avoid that particular food for the time being. If the change is slightly less, say seven, eight or nine beats per minute, it might not be necessary to avoid that food completely but you should certainly treat it with respect, eating it no more frequently than every four days; even then, you might find that you feel better if you don't eat it at all. If the change is less than seven beats per minute and you experience no symptoms, you may assume that it is safe to reintroduce that food to your diet.

You can check out several foods, or families of foods, in this way, moving straight on to five days' avoidance of the next foods to be tested. If at any stage you experience really severe symptoms, take lots of vitamin C and, as an emergency measure, mix half a teaspoon of salt with half a teaspoon of bicarbonate of soda in a tumbler of warm water and drink it down quickly – followed by something more palatable! This should start to reduce the symptoms in half an hour or so.

This is about the most reliable (and easily the cheapest!) form of allergy-testing available, so it is well worth the trouble it takes to do it. If you are not sure how to take your pulse, put the fingers of one hand flat across the inside of your opposite wrist (this hand with its palm facing up is probably easier), pressing slightly below the thumb.

Alternatively, press the tips of your fingers into the front of your neck, towards the side, just under your jawbone.

Among the most common foods to cause an intolerance are grains; it might be a specific grain which is causing problems, or it might be all the grains which contain gluten (wheat, oats, rye and barley). Sometimes, there is a reaction to just one or possibly two of the gluten grains (wheat or oats sensitivity are very common) but in this situation there is not an all-out gluten intolerance. Surprisingly, perhaps, even if you have to avoid *all* the gluten grains, there are still several others which you should be able to eat – maize, millet, buckwheat, whole rice, quinoa. You will find many recipes in this book which are marked 'gluten-free', as well as a section at the back of the book. Some practitioners believe that all candida sufferers are better without gluten, but I have not found this necessary unless an intolerance is found to the whole gluten family.

Very often, it becomes possible in due course to reintroduce the culprit foods, although it might first be necessary to take additional steps to heal the 'leaky gut' which has allowed the situation to arise. There is usually not much point in attempting this before candida is fairly well under control; it is rather like applying wood-filler to a beam which is full of woodworm holes when the worms are still active. They will simply pop up around the edges! The approach needed therefore is to avoid the foods in order to keep a load off the immune system until candida is under control and then, when antifungals are no longer needed, take specific supplements to heal the intestinal lining. At this stage, improvement often comes after just a couple of months, but there are various ways of helping to heal the gut wall so you would be well advised to consult a nutritionist for help with this situation.

When there is a total intolerance to gluten or to cow's milk (another common culprit), this sometimes has to be accepted as a lifetime situation. This type of intolerance is not due to a leaky gut but to an enzyme deficiency; your body simply doesn't make the enzymes necessary to digest those specific foods. However, the situation is not as bad as it seems because, once you are well, you can take enzyme supplements when it is impossible to avoid gluten or dairy foods, such as when eating away from home; but this is not something you would want to do all the time so it is better to adjust to good alternatives, as discussed on page 259.

Low Blood Sugar (Hypoglycaemia)

Low blood sugar causes many unpleasant symptoms, such as fatigue, depression and headache, and is very often a problem in people with yeast-infection. Let me explain.

Imagine a graph drawn across a page. If you are suffering from low blood sugar, every time you eat sugar or a food which quickly turns to glucose once digested (like white flour or white rice), the level of glucose in your blood will rush to a high point on the graph. If it stayed up there, you would have a condition of high blood sugar, or diabetes, so the body very cleverly does something to bring the level down. The pancreas receives a signal to release some insulin, which brings the sugar level down but allows it to drop to a low point on the graph. At this stage, you will probably feel your worst in whichever ways it affects you in particular. You might feel dizzy and faint, or have a headache, or feel irritable or depressed, or just plain exhausted. So you reach for something that will give you a 'lift', something which you know from experience will pick you up quite quickly. It might be tea or coffee, or a biscuit, or some chocolate, or a can of cola, a glass of beer or a gin and tonic.

Very soon the headache has gone, you feel soothed and able to cope once more – but unfortunately it doesn't last. This is because your raised sugar level has triggered the release of more insulin, so that once again the line on the graph has plummeted down to a low point. The pancreas becomes trigger-happy and over-reacts, so the line on the graph goes from high to low to high to low and so on, right across the page. Those parts of the body which are trying desperately to control the situation become increasingly exhausted, and the situation gets worse. Eventually, the pancreas becomes so exhausted that it is unable to produce more insulin, which means that the sugar in your blood remains at a high level with nothing to bring it down – and that is a common cause of late-onset adult diabetes.

What needs to be done is to change the line on your graph from peaks and troughs to a gentle, undulating curve of slight ups and downs. You can do this by eating foods which slowly release just small amounts of sugar into your blood, and also by eating frequently so that you 'catch' the line before it drops too low. The most helpful foods are complex carbohydrates (whole grains and vegetables – also fruit, but not if you're on the anti-candida diet!) and good quality protein (low fat natural yoghurt, cottage cheese, chicken, fish, eggs, tofu, beans and pulses). You also need the right supplements in your programme. For instance, vitamin B_3 and the mineral chromium help the liver to release a substance called Glucose Tolerance Factor which makes insulin more potent. Vitamins B and C give support to the adrenal glands while things get back to normal. Improving glucose tolerance (correcting low blood sugar) takes a load off all the parts of the body which are trying to control the situation, so that they are no longer exhausted and may be restored to health and efficiency. You can almost hear your adrenals and your pancreas breathe an enormous sigh of relief! If low blood sugar seems to be a problem to you, your nutritionist will certainly take account of it in your diet and supplement programme.

There is no reason why your energy levels and stamina should not become more stable and reliable than they have ever been before.

Stress

One factor I would like to discuss here is the role played by stress in encouraging an overgrowth of candida and in slowing down the rate at which it is overcome. This is because stress triggers the production of adrenaline which in turn triggers the release of the body's sugar stores, thus enabling candida to have a bean-feast! However, adrenaline copes only with short-term stress, so ongoing or protracted stress means that the body needs more help, and this is provided in the form of two other adrenal hormones, cortisol and DHEA. Cortisol is meant to be produced in a regular daily cycle which starts high in the morning and ends low at night but, if extra is needed to help the body cope with long-term stress, the 'body-clock' goes haywire. This has many adverse effects including an inability to experience refreshing sleep, energy slumps during the day, lack of temperature control, poor skin healing and weakened immunity. The situation becomes a vicious circle because long-term illness in itself is stressful, and inflammation of any type also places a load on the adrenal stress hormones.

It can be helpful in this situation to undertake a diagnostic test (through Diagnostech laboratory in Wales, UK, also in USA, available through nutritionists), using saliva specimens collected at set times during the day, which show the levels and behaviour of the main stress hormones compared with a normal reference range. With this information, it becomes possible to support both cortisol and DHEA in whichever ways are necessary by taking appropriate nutritional supplements and, in addition, by knowing at which times of day to take them in order to manipulate the irregular daily cycle back to a normal reference range. The problem is that, even when a stressful situation abates, the adrenal stress hormones stay over-adapted and they need specific help to get back on the right track. This can take a few months to achieve, but the effort is well worthwhile in terms of increased immune function and victory over candida alone. And of course it must still be remembered that, even though a diagnostic test to show the levels and behaviour of adrenal stress hormones is extremely helpful, it is also essential to sort out your lifestyle and problems in practical terms as far as you can, in order to minimize the effects of ongoing stress.

If you are being advised by a nutritionist and if you have a problem at any time, you should tell your practitioner so that the situation may be assessed and a decision made as to how best to help you.

Vaginal Thrush

A very common problem with women is vaginal thrush, which shows itself in various forms from heavy discharge to irritation or severe inflammation. This condition will eventually respond to the regime which is sorting out the situation from the inside, but it is also helpful to use an antifungal cream. I recommend a product which is able to penetrate the tissues with friendly bacteria and ensure that the environment has the correct acidity to destroy candida and encourage the good guys. In addition, an ointment or pessaries containing tea tree oil are frequently found to be helpful. However, the situation will almost certainly not clear completely until the balance of microbes in the intestines has first of all been corrected, and even then it might take some time. It is the same with skin conditions like eczema; the balance of microbes on the surface of the skin or mucous membranes reflects the balance in the intestines but is three months behind, so that even when the situation is fully corrected internally, you might have to wait another twelve weeks before external conditions finally start to clear up.

Chapter 5

How Long?

So, how long will it take to get fully well? How long is a piece of string? I'm afraid it is quite impossible to say because each person is unique. It depends on how much candida overgrowth you have, how long you have had it, the strength of your immune system, how much stress is in your life, how many allergies need to be discovered, how toxic your liver has become, etc., etc. I have known a very few people become fully well in the first three months. For a larger number, it has taken six months, and for even more, nine months or a year. For those who have been severely ill for a considerable period of time, it has taken even longer, yet even these clients have known that they were moving along the right lines, with a considerable degree of improvement after a year. Perhaps the greatest number of people, including many who were really quite ill to start with, take somewhere between nine months and a year to have a full return of energy, able to return to work and live a normal, symptom-free life. Ten or eleven months of moving forward even slowly is better than ten months of standing still or going backwards!

However ill you are to start with, and however long it is going to take you to recover, I hope you will find the motivation you need to stay on the regime until all the candida overgrowths in your body are fully under control. Of course, if you have found a helpful nutritionist, you will receive ongoing advice and support, but in the end you are the one who must take responsibility for your health.

I constantly find that no matter how much I warn people about die-off reaction, either they don't believe me or they fail to take it in so that, when they start to get what seems like a flare-up of old symptoms or they feel achy and depressed, they forget that I warned them this might happen and become really worried. Or, if they do remember, they still say, 'I didn't know it was going to be as bad as this!' You need to get it firmly fixed in your mind before it happens, so that you can hold on to the understanding that die-off symptoms are actually a very good thing. They mean that candida is being destroyed. Die-off is just a temporary phase, and you can control it by being sensible about the level of antifungals that you take and by supporting your liver in its work of detoxification. Die-off often comes in surges, as candida is destroyed in different areas of your body. Each experience of die-off is not a disappointing setback but a welcome step forward.

There is no easy way of bringing candida under control. Most people have to go through this process of die-off reaction to some extent, but it really does not have to be worse than you can bear because you are the one who is in control and in a position to regulate the levels of antifungals which you take. Some people push on regardless (particularly young men with a macho image!), taking high levels of antifungals much too soon and getting themselves into a sorry state by thinking they can speed up the whole process. Well, they soon find out that it can't be done. Toxins from dead yeast have to be eliminated via the liver, and there is no point in overloading it. It really is best to take things slowly but surely, just as fast as your body can cope with eliminating the extra toxins being released by dead yeast. You only experience die-off symptoms when you are destroying candida more quickly than your liver can deal with its toxins – so find ways of helping your liver but, in any case, take it slowly.

If you decide to go ahead and follow the four-point plan, I hope you will see it as an adventure and not as a hardship. Just think how good it will be to feel well again. And think, too, how much you will have learned along the way – how to exercise self-discipline, determination and patience, and how to enjoy eating healthily for all the years ahead!

In my practice, each consultation allows time in the following three months for the client to telephone and ask questions or check out any points of confusion, whether about diet, supplements or symptoms. Fighting candida is an experience which needs to be shared, whenever possible, with someone who understands what is happening and can encourage you along the way. The proof of the pudding (if you'll forgive the expression!) is that one-time candida sufferers are able to support and encourage other 'yeasties' as they go through the process of overcoming candidiasis. If you can envisage doing that for someone else before very long, it will give point and value to your own experience as you step forward into the four-point plan.

So, the place to start is with the anti-candida diet. In Chapter 6 you will find the guidelines which I give to all my yeasty clients. I tell them to read the diet sheet at home and get over their initial heart attack! After that, they can contact my office to sort out any queries they might have about what is and is not allowed, and discuss the question of what is left to eat!

As you study the guidelines, they will probably come as a shock at first. For most people, it means making radical changes to their present eating habits but, having read through the basic rules, look at them again and you will begin to see that life might still be worth living, after all.

And that, of course, is where the remainder of this book comes in. A quick flick through the recipe pages will show you that in fact the anti-candida diet provides food fit for a king. If you are feeling the least bit sorry for yourself just at this moment at the thought of all those foods you are having to give up, believe me, you are in for a real surprise!

You have possibly come across other books which recommend diets that are either more lenient or more stringent than this one. I can only say that I have never yet seen a 'yeasty' person become fully well on a more lenient diet, particularly whilst eating even the smallest amount of fruit. For the time being, fruit has to go. Meanwhile, plenty of salads and fresh vegetables together with a good supplement programme will make sure that you are not deficient in vitamins and minerals. On the other hand, it is pretty impossible to stick to some diets which are stricter than this one, and that causes feelings of failure on top of everything else.

This is a diet which I *know* will achieve its objective of starving candida to death. Not only will it help to bring your symptoms under control in the next few weeks and months but it will also help to change your taste buds so that your personal preference in future will be for healthy foods, keeping you in the best possible health for the rest of your life, and in particular ensuring that candida in your body stays firmly under control.

Chapter 6

The Anti-candida Diet
(to be used as part of the four-point plan)

Foods to Avoid

☹ **SUGAR**, in all its forms, and food containing sugar. This includes brown or white sugar, demerara, molasses, syrup, honey, malt, chocolate and all other forms of confectionery, icing, marzipan, ice cream, desserts and puddings, cakes and biscuits, soft drinks including squash and all canned drinks, tinned fruit in syrup, etc. Check all tins and packets for hidden sugar – even some frozen and canned vegetables! Types of sugar include fructose, lactose, maltose, sucrose and dextrose.

☹ **YEAST** – all food containing it or derived from it. This includes bread, food coated in breadcrumbs, Marmite, Vecon, Bovril, Bisto, Oxo, etc., citric acid, monosodium glutamate, vitamin tablets (unless the label specifically states 'yeast-free'), pizza bases and most makes of pitta bread. Beware of commercial wrapped bread which claims to have no added yeast if it has been made with sourdough or sprouted grains because these products have been fermented and contain their own naturally-produced yeasts.

☹ **REFINED GRAINS** – white flour, granary flour (which is white flour with malt and added whole grains), white rice, white pasta, cornflour (cornstarch), custard powder, cornflakes and cereals (unless 'whole grain' or 'wholemeal' is stated).

☹ **MALTED PRODUCTS** – some cereals (e.g. Weetabix), some crispbreads, granary bread, malted drinks like Ovaltine, Horlicks and Caro.

☹ **ANYTHING FERMENTED** – vinegar and foods containing it (ketchups, pickles, salad cream, baked beans), also soy sauce, sourdough bread, ginger beer, cider, beer and wine. In fact all alcohol, including spirits, acts as a stimulant which triggers the release of your sugar stores.

☹ **COW'S MILK** and most milk products, including cream and most cheeses. (See following notes about yoghurt, cottage cheese and butter.)

☹ **FRESH FRUIT**, raw, stewed, made into jam or juice. (Pure fruit juice is virtually 'straight' fructose and often also very high in mould.) Freshly-squeezed lemon juice is allowed in salad dressing, mineral water, etc.

☹ **DRIED FRUIT**, including prunes and the fruit in muesli. N.B. Figs or dates are used to sweeten some health drinks (e.g. Caro, Bambu, Nocaff).

☹ **NUTS,** unless freshly cracked, because of mould. Avoid peanuts completely, even in their shells (monkey nuts) because they are very high in mould. Avoid peanut butter for this reason.

☹ **SMOKED OR CURED** fish and meat, including ham, bacon (even unsmoked is still cured) and smoked salmon, smoked mackerel, smoked haddock.

☹ **MUSHROOMS**, which are a fungus (so are truffles).

☹ **TEA AND COFFEE** – even decaffeinated, because they still contain other stimulants. Also avoid **HOT CHOCOLATE**.

☹ **COLA DRINKS AND LUCOZADE** – they both contain caffeine, as do **BEECHAM'S POWDERS** and **SOME PAINKILLERS** (e.g. Anadin, Phensic, Panadol Extra).

☹ **ARTIFICIAL SWEETENERS**, which have been found to feed candida just as effectively as sugar, and in any case keep your sweet tooth alive.

☹ **PRESERVATIVES**, including citric acid, which are frequently derived from yeasts and in any case introduce chemicals to the body. (N.B. Sausages, even without preservatives, are high in animal fat and refined cereal.)

☹ **HOT SPICES AND CURRIES** because they destroy friendly bacteria in the intestines.

Worried? You needn't be. Coming next are lots of enjoyable alternatives.

PLEASE NOTE: Some medications encourage the growth of yeast, especially antibiotics and steroids (including creams and inhalers, the contraceptive pill and HRT) and NSAIDs (non-steroidal anti-inflammatory drugs). Also, rid your home of mould or damp – regularly clean around double-glazed windows – and get rid of all your house plants; mould from the soil becomes airborne and could be keeping you ill.

Foods to Enjoy

☺ **YEAST-FREE SODA BREAD** made with wholewheat flour or other grains (*see recipes following*). Some bakers will make a batch for your freezer.

☺ **RICE CAKES** (may be lightly toasted), **OAT CAKES** (malt-free), **ORIGINAL or SESAME RYVITA**, **WHOLEWHEAT CRISPBREADS** (read labels carefully).

☺ **PASTRY** made with wholemeal flour, oatmeal and sunflower or olive oil, in proportions of 3:2:2. Make very moist with plenty of water and dust well with flour before rolling.

☺ **SOYA MILK** or **RICE MILK** as milk alternatives. (Different makes of soya milk have very different flavours.)

☺ **BUTTER** (unsalted) for spreading or cooking; otherwise for cooking use extra virgin olive oil.

☺ **UNHYDROGENATED MARGARINE**. Read the labels carefully to make sure you pick the right ones. Avoid those with citric acid.

☺ **COLD-PRESSED OILS**: sunflower, safflower, linseed, as salad dressing mixed with lemon juice, and with an egg for mayonnaise.

☺ **NATURAL YOGHURT Low-fat, natural, unflavoured**: try it for dessert or breakfast with lecithin granules or a mixture of seeds, or with a cereal like whole puffed rice. Spread it on top of wholewheat lasagne dishes before baking, or flavour with mint as a dip.

☺ **COTTAGE CHEESE** as a spread or a filler for your jacket potato or with salad.

☺ **BREAKFASTS**: home-made muesli with oatflakes and other whole grains mixed with seeds, soaked in water and eaten with soya milk, rice milk or natural yoghurt; Shredded Wheat with soya milk or rice milk; puffed oats, puffed wheat or puffed rice or Kashi (mixed whole grains) with soya milk or rice milk; porridge made with water or soya milk, sprinkled with cinnamon or nutmeg and eaten with yoghurt; egg (boiled, poached or scrambled) eaten with wholewheat soda bread or toast and butter; rice cakes with cottage cheese and sliced tomato; slices of tinned pease pudding with tomato, grilled or heated in the microwave – and many more besides!

☺ **MAIN MEALS**: try to find a butcher selling free-range chickens and 'organic' lean meat to avoid hormones and antibiotics (lamb and rabbit are less likely to be affected), but don't forget that red meat has inflammatory properties. Enjoy any type of fish, but oily fish is particularly beneficial (herrings, sardines, mackerel, pilchards, salmon, tuna and trout). Combine a grain with a pulse for a complete vegetarian protein, e.g., bean and vegetable pie or crumble, rice or bulgar with chickpeas in a tomato or soya milk and herb sauce, whole wheat spaghetti or brown rice pasta twirls with brown lentils, tomatoes and onions.

- ☺ **FRESH VEGETABLES** of all types, steamed. Aim to have a plateful of **SALAD,** including **TOMATOES**, every day.
- ☺ **AVOCADOS** are good filled with cottage cheese and humus, or yoghurt with tomato purée, and topped with slices of cucumber.
- ☺ **LEMONS**: apart from avocados, the only fruit allowed. If adding a slice to your drinks, scrub the peel well to remove traces of mould. Use lemon juice for salad dressing, for a yoghurt sauce with casseroled chicken and for squeezing over your fish.
- ☺ **SEEDS AND FRESHLY CRACKED NUTS** (not peanuts) make nutritious snacks. Choose seeds from sunflower, pumpkin, flax and sesame. Keep in the fridge. N.B. Shelled nuts have unseen mould.
- ☺ **HERBS** of all kinds, fresh or dried, add interesting variations in flavour to your meals.
- ☺ **MILD SPICES** also add interest (cinnamon, coriander, cumin, turmeric, etc.) but avoid the hot ones, especially chilli.
- ☺ **HOT DRINKS**: Barleycup and any type of herb tea or fruit tea provided it has no added citric acid or malt or artificial flavourings or colourings. Rooibosch tastes closest to 'ordinary' tea. Hot tomato juice makes a nice winter warmer. Roasted dandelion root 'coffee' (avoid added lactose) tastes good and is wonderful for detoxifying your liver.
- ☺ **COLD DRINKS**: filtered or bottled water, still or sparkling, with added ice and lemon not only looks good but is refreshing and delicious. (As an alternative to buying bottles of sparkling mineral water, use a filter jug and a soda siphon.) Chilled tomato juice (no citric acid or vinegar) is good as a 'starter', and iced fruit teas (no citric acid or malt) make a tasty alternative to fruit juice in summer. Try whisking yoghurt with sparkling mineral water and adding mint leaves or vanilla essence.

Lactose-containing Foods

Lactose is a natural sugar which occurs in milk and therefore in milk products like cheese and butter. Because it is a form of sugar, candida will thrive on it as much as on ordinary table sugar. My general advice is that lactose should be strictly avoided, although a couple of very slight exceptions may be made if people are responding well to the rest of the programme. Some people react to dairy produce in any case, because their immune systems cannot tolerate its protein content, so by avoiding these items at least until candida is under control they prevent an unnecessary load being placed on the immune system. For those who do not have a dairy intolerance, I allow the use of low-fat natural yoghurt, a small amount of butter and also cottage cheese; but, if progress is not sufficiently encouraging, I might recommend complete avoidance of even this small amount of dairy produce for the time being. Cottage cheese is roughly two per cent lactose and, although this amount makes no difference to most people, to a few others it is sufficient to hold back progress. The small amount of butter needed for spreading on soda bread or rice cakes contains only a little lactose, but even this might prove to be too much in some stubborn cases. In any case, animal fat has inflammatory properties so if you suffer from aches and pains or hormonal problems, you would benefit more from eating unhydrogenated margarine (*see Chapter 7*).

Goat's milk has only slightly less lactose than cow's milk. Whether or not you can get away with using it depends on the progress you make with the rest of the programme. I once thought it was 'safe' to use goat's milk on the anti-candida regime but I now believe it is best to use only soya milk (beware of added fruit juice) or oat milk (ditto) or rice milk made from organic wholegrain rice.

In view of this concern about lactose, I am often asked why yoghurt is allowed. The answer is that in yoghurt most of the lactose is already digested by an enzyme called lactase, produced by live bacteria. Lactose then becomes lactic acid, which is why yoghurt has a characteristic 'sharp' flavour; it has lost the natural sweetness of milk. Apart from this, yoghurt contains friendly bacteria which happen to be the same sort that are needed in our intestines. This fact would seem to outweigh the possible problems caused by any small amount of remaining lactose; even so, if one of my clients is not making satisfactory progress, I recommend coming off yoghurt for a while to see if it makes any difference. In addition, any cow's milk product has a tendency to cause a build-up of mucus, so if you suffer from catarrh or sinusitis, it would be a very good idea to avoid yoghurt and cottage cheese for a while, even if you do not have an actual intolerance to dairy produce. However, the main advantage of being able to include yoghurt in your diet is that it makes a very easy dessert!

Most cheeses contain only a small amount of lactose but they have been fermented and contain some mould (even though they might look very clean and yellow), so all types of cheese other than cottage cheese must be avoided for the time being.

Special Note: Don't be fooled into buying cartons of milk labelled 'Low Lactose'; it still does contain some lactose and also glucose.

So now you have the basic rules for the anti-candida diet, but it is also important to know some general rules about wise and healthy eating in order to build your all-round health, and these are included in the next chapter.

I really hope you enjoy getting into the diet. You can adapt many recipes from other books simply by changing from white flour to wholewheat flour (or wholemeal – it's the same thing). If you are underweight and afraid of losing more, this certainly need not happen from the point of view of calorie-intake because you may eat as much as you like of the foods which are allowed – in fact, if you are one of those lucky people who doesn't put on half a stone at the sight of a slice of bread, you may eat wholewheat soda bread, carrot cake, dumplings, Yorkshire pudding, porridge and filling root vegetables to your heart's content!

On the other hand, overweight people are usually very encouraged to find that they lose weight more easily than ever before. The reason for this is that, when we eat some food regularly to which our immune systems have an intolerance, the body tries to cope with the situation by retaining fluids to dilute the offending food, and this fluid retention causes weight gain. If you can pinpoint and stop eating the culprit food, the body is able to off-load the excess fluid and, with it, some excess weight. Since most people with an overgrowth of yeast in their bodies will have a sensitivity to yeast in their diet, every time they have eaten a slice of yeasted bread or had some cheese or yeasty gravy, and every time they have drunk some wine or beer (both of which are high in yeast), their bodies will have held on to some fluid to dilute it. This means that when they embark on the anti-candida diet which avoids all those foods, excess weight is very often shed quickly and easily, without the need to reduce calories.

If they lose some excess weight in the first month but then it sticks, this is a strong indication that there is another food which is still being allowed in the anti-candida diet but to which they have a specific intolerance; it might be wheat, or potatoes, or almost any other food which they eat on a frequent basis, and this is where the pulse test is helpful to clarify the situation (see page 34). Find the offender, and more weight will be lost.

Once you are well, it would be foolish and dangerous to throw the anti-candida diet overboard too soon and to forget all you have learned about healthy eating. It is first of all necessary to carry out a diet-relax experiment for a month to make sure that even healthy yeasty foods will not re-encourage candida. It involves trying some crisp peeled fruit (apple, pear) on two days in the first week, then adding some wholewheat yeasted bread twice in the second week, some Edam or Gouda cheese twice in the third week and semi-skimmed cow's milk twice in the fourth, so that by the last week of the month you are eating all four types of food twice in the week. Don't be tempted to try fruits other than apples and pears at this stage; others are extremely high in fructose and some (oranges, plums, grapes, melon) are high in natural yeast. And don't forget that this experiment must only last for a month.

After that, even if all has gone well and you have experienced no flare-up of any of your old symptoms, you need to forget the bread, milk, cheese and fruit again and stay within the guidelines of the diet for a whole year more. This is necessary in order to consolidate what has just been achieved in establishing a new healthy balance of micro-organisms in the intestines, which takes *a further year* on the anti-candida diet. This follow-up year once you are feeling well pays dividends over and over again, and means it is virtually certain that you will then be free to enjoy fruit, yeasted wholewheat bread, cheese, etc., without fear of re-encouraging your resident candida to overgrow and thrive.

However, it is also virtually certain that if you were to return to sugar, stimulants and the type of junk foods which helped to make you ill in the first place, your resident candida would quickly make its presence felt once more; it is not a question that once you've had yeast infection you are never totally free of it, simply that you would be doing all the things necessary to encourage it just as you did in the first place!

During the follow-up year, you may in fact have just a little more freedom on a very occasional basis if you are eating out or away from home (provided you relax the diet in *sensible* ways); but, by keeping to the diet for a further year on a day-to-day basis, you will be consolidating your new-found health. If you start breaking the diet at home, it is so easy to go overboard – especially if you seem to be getting away with it – but in fact you run a constant risk of encouraging candida to thrive once more. It happens all too easily; I know because, in ignorance at the time, I did it myself and suffered the consequences, and it is very much harder to start all over again for a second time, believe me.

My real hope is that you will see the diet not just as a ploy to rob you of all the foods and drinks you most enjoy – something to be rebelled against at the first opportunity – but as a means of re-educating your mind and your taste buds to appreciate food which is both good to eat and good for your body. Once you have lost your 'sweet tooth' (and you will, because you were not born with it), there is no point in encouraging it back again. Sugar is an anti-nutrient; in other words, it uses up essential nutrients simply to help the body deal with it. It does us no good whatsoever. If you have read my explanation of low blood sugar on page 35, you will realize just how much of a fallacy it is that we need sugar for energy. I hope that other junk foods will also remain a thing of the past; I am sure they will, once you have learned to appreciate the vastly superior flavour of natural wholefoods. There is simply no comparison! Just allow time for your taste buds to come alive; until now, they have been deadened by sugar. And if you think that food without salt lacks flavour, just wait for your nutritional status to improve. A craving for salt suggests a zinc deficiency and, as you will now be getting zinc in your supplement programme, before long you will discover that natural foods have far more flavour than you ever believed possible.

You have the opportunity to learn – possibly for the first time, as I did – how to eat the foods which your body requires as fuel for its machinery. More than that, you have the opportunity to learn how to *enjoy* eating them, and in so doing you will be laying down the best possible foundation for your future health.

Chapter 7

General Guidelines for Healthy Eating

The following changes to your general eating habits, as well as the specific requirements of the anti-candida diet, will help you to obtain and absorb nutrients, revitalize your body and speed up the health-promoting benefits of your supplement programme. The principles behind these recommendations are in accordance with the teaching of the Institute for Optimum Nutrition in London.

1) Make sure that at least half of your diet consists of alkaline-forming foods: all vegetables, sprouted seeds, yoghurt (natural, unsweetened), buckwheat and freshly-cracked almonds.

2) The rest of your diet should consist of acid-forming foods such as whole grains, beans and pulses, nuts (freshly cracked), seeds, free-range eggs, cottage cheese, fish and poultry. Avoid refined grains like white flour and white rice as these quickly turn to sugar in the blood and have been deprived of many beneficial nutrients and fibre, causing an imbalance of vitamins and minerals and encouraging constipation.

3) Eat as many raw vegetables as possible. Cooking destroys vitamins and breaks down the fibre in food. Have a large plate of salad at least once a day.

4) The best proportion of food at *every* meal and *every* snack is **one-third** good quality protein (fish, chicken, yoghurt, cottage cheese, beans, pulses, tofu) to **two-thirds** complex carbohydrates (all vegetables and whole grains). This gives you the best energy and the most efficient metabolism by helping to regulate blood sugar, support your adrenals and strengthen immunity.

5) When using oils other than for cooking (i.e. for salad dressings, spreads, mayonnaise), use cold-pressed (or unrefined) sunflower, sesame, safflower or flax (linseed)

oils. You will also derive helpful oils by eating seeds as snacks (try pumpkin) or sprinkled on your breakfast, ground or whole. Do NOT use margarine which states 'hydrogenated', even if it also claims to be high in polyunsaturates! The process of hydrogenation makes the oils more harmful to the body than saturated animal fats, so look for the word 'unhydrogenated' on the tub before you buy it. The best oils produce prostaglandins which are needed for healthy hormones and skin. They also reduce inflammation.

6) Avoid frying; grill or bake instead. If you do fry, use cold-pressed, extra virgin olive oil or a small amount of butter (which is actually safer at very high temperatures than sunflower oil) and cook for as short a time as possible. Cold-pressed sunflower oil may be used at baking temperatures (it makes excellent pastry) but is damaging if used at higher temperatures.

7) Increase fish and poultry (free-range, to avoid antibiotics and hormones). Reduce red meats like beef, pork and lamb and other high-fat foods. Even lean meat is 75 per cent fat. Among other things, they cause inflammation and so encourage aches and pains.

8) Increase vegetarian sources of protein. A complete protein is made by having a meal which combines *a grain* with *a pulse* (*see Anti-candida Diet Main Meals*, *page 44*).

9) The essential fatty acid from oily fish is good for you, producing prostaglandins (hormone-like substances) which are beneficial for the health of your heart and arteries, so helping to reduce high blood pressure. They also reduce inflammation.

10) The ideal intake of water is about 2 litres (3½ pints) daily. However, a diet which has plenty of raw vegetables will supply some of this, since these foods are 90 per cent water. We should therefore aim at drinking 1–1½ litres (1¾–2½ pints) of water a day, taken as filtered or mineral water or in herb teas or fruit teas. Filter jugs are a good idea but be sure to change the filter regularly. You might even consider a plumbed-in filter system; some are excellent, both in terms of improved flavour of the water and of purity.

11) Avoid foods with added salt. Don't add salt to your cooking and, if you must add something at the table, use Lo-Salt, which has more potassium than sodium. If you think your food lacks flavour without salt, this probably means that your body is zinc-deficient. Add flavour with herbs and mild spices.

12) Avoid artificial additives and preservatives, which means avoiding processed or 'fast' foods. Also avoid artificial sweeteners; they upset the chemical balance of the body and can even cause depression. In any case, they keep your sweet tooth alive, and that is something you are definitely better without!

13) Smoking not only causes damage to your lungs and arteries but also directly interferes with the absorption of many nutrients, causing nutritional deficiencies and imbalances which weaken your immune system and give rise to other health problems.

Stimulants

The restriction on tea, coffee, sugar, cola and alcohol found in the anti-candida diet guidelines (Chapter 6) is just as relevant to a general healthy diet as it is to an anti-candida programme. They are all stressors, which means that they stimulate the adrenal glands to react in just the same way as they do to psychological stress; in the short term, adrenaline is released and, in the long term, additional cortisol is released, causing the body clock to go haywire and other adverse effects, including a shutdown of digestive processes, excess glucose in the bloodstream, increased heart rate and raised blood pressure.

In this process, nutrients are used up and resistance to infection becomes low. With too much stimulation, the adrenal glands become exhausted and need more and more stimulation to make them work. This creates a craving for more stimulants – sugar, tea, coffee, cola, alcohol – and so addictions set in. The effect on the body of stimulants is exactly the same as the effect of stress – whether anger, fear, worry or frustration – and both have long-term harmful effects. Even stress is addictive!

Apart from their role as stimulants, tea and coffee have an amazing number of other harmful effects. For instance, caffeine causes us to lose chromium, which is needed to help stabilize blood sugar levels. Caffeine actually increases a craving for sugar, and caffeine and tannin (in tea) deplete the body of iron, potassium, zinc and B vitamins. Coffee – even decaffeinated – increases the secretion of acid in the stomach, causing problems in the digestive tract and leading to malabsorption of nutrients.

If you find it hard to believe that you are actually addicted to one of these substances – whether tea, coffee, chocolate, cola or sugar – just see what happens when you decide to come off it! You will almost certainly get a headache for a couple of days because you will be going through symptoms of drug-withdrawal.

It is obvious that all stimulants put a strain on the body, even in someone who is reasonably healthy. For a 'yeasty' person, battling against an overgrowth of Candida albicans, it is even more obvious that these and other stimulants must be totally avoided. When you start to feel well, you will honestly wonder why you ever bothered to put such rubbish in your body!

Chapter 8

Using the Recipes

Many of the recipes in both the first and second editions of this book were contributed by my clients. They were accompanied by comments that they were good to eat, easy to prepare – and also that they had proved to be popular with family and friends, which of course is very important.

As recipes arrived in the post for the first edition, I was struck by two things. First, that people who had originally thought the diet was going to be a bleak experience had come up with a great deal of creative talent – and that's not easy when you have a muzzy head and all the other yeasty symptoms! The other realization was that recipes were coming in from people with very varied energy levels. Some were able to go out to work and still manage to entertain their friends; others were struggling through the day with a very limited amount of energy; and still others spent all their days in bed, relying on friends or relations to look after them. The recipes they sent reflected their state of health and the requirements and limitations of their lifestyle.

People in the last two categories would obviously find a book of recipes aimed at catering for 'yeasty' dinner parties to be unhelpful and depressing in the extreme, yet those who want to entertain their friends within the limitations of the anti-candida diet need more helpful suggestions than to offer their guests a bowl of yoghurt with seeds on top!

That was how the idea came that the recipes in this book should have a star rating, the number of stars denoting the simplicity of the recipe or, to put it another way, the amount of energy required to prepare it. For recipes requiring the least energy, the rating is one star (*). Basic baking and recipes using a moderate amount of energy have been given two stars (**). The really tricky stuff – meals you could serve for a dinner party which take a fair amount of preparation – have been given three stars (***). In fact, there are only a few recipes in this third category, because many of the dishes with one or two stars could be used for entertaining in any case, and there is no point in expending energy needlessly.

I have called the three categories:

*   Surviving
**   Reviving
***   Thriving

I am sure you don't need anyone to tell you which of those three describes *your* situation right now!

All kitchen tasks can be made a great deal easier with the right equipment, so some recipes which have been given two stars (**) would make the one star (*) grade if you had a food processor, for instance. Obviously, it is not possible to come up with a hard-and-fast rule for deciding on categories, but it is a fact that you expend much less energy if you have a few gadgets. Let's have a look at some which are well worth using if you have them, or possibly worth investing in.

1) Little collapsible steamer trays made of stainless steel save energy and strength if you have weak arms because you don't have to strain the vegetables over a sink; but their real asset is that they produce vegetables which are crisp and un-mushy, well-coloured and full of nutrients. They fit any size saucepan and are quite cheap to buy.

2) A liquidizer or blender which has a grinder attachment is fairly inexpensive and invaluable for making vegetable purée for soups and stocks, and also for grinding seeds to make savoury spreads.

3) A pepper mill for grinding black peppercorns is good because pepper which is freshly ground is far less likely to harbour mould than pre-ground pepper. Research has shown that pepper pots can contain really high levels of mould.

4) Rather more expensive (but something I now wouldn't be without) is a food processor. I was given one on my 50th birthday, and it revolutionized my pastry-making! It may also be used for making cakes, blending mayonnaise, grating carrots … the list is endless.

5) For people with only a small amount of energy which possibly comes at certain times of day, a slow-cooker is a real boon. Prepare the meal whilst you have some strength, put it all in the pot, forget it, and it will be ready to eat some hours later.

6) Pressure cookers come into their own when cooking beans, which otherwise take a long time. They are also useful when you want a complete meal ready in a short time, although they are pretty heavy to handle. If you are buying a new one, save up for the stainless steel variety and avoid aluminium.

7) Stainless steel or heatproof glass saucepans are not only more healthy than aluminium or non-stick (both of which release traces of toxic substances), but they are also so much easier to clean.

8) A microwave oven saves time and energy. Porridge cooks straight in the dish, so saving a sticky pan; onions 'sweat' really quickly when you're preparing the base for a meal; and you can blind-bake a 25cm/10-inch pastry case in just six minutes. Fish and vegetables straight from the freezer cook in a very short time and have a good flavour.

9) Casserole oven dishes, large and small, are a great help because you can put the food in a low-heat oven and leave it to cook very slowly. Also, having dishes with lids on keeps the oven clean and avoids another job.

10) There must be very few families these days without a refrigerator, but if you happen to be one of them, you really should not eat food left over from the previous day because it will have started to gather mould. Even with a refrigerator, you should aim to eat food as soon after cooking as possible.

11) A freezer is a tremendous help because it enables you to make two meals at a time and freeze one for another day. You can also freeze chicken or vegetable stock in yoghurt tubs ready to use, and batches of soda bread or scones – all ways of making life easier on days when you have less energy. It also helps by making shopping trips less frequent.

There is nothing on the above list which is absolutely essential but, if you do happen to own any of these items, learn to think ahead and make the best use of them.

At the end of the book is a section giving ideas for packed lunches, including some children's favourites, and another section giving ideas for those who are suffering from specific food intolerances which need to be taken into account for the time being – fat, wheat, gluten or even all the grains.

Finally, there is a section giving menus for a period of two weeks, together with a shopping list of the foods you will need to buy. This is not intended to be one of those menu-outlines which you are supposed to follow religiously day-by-day and meal-by-meal, but simply an attempt to help you get to grips with a new way of eating. The best way to use the plan is to 'mix and match' to suit yourself.

So, now you can start cooking and eating. Just think – not only will you enjoy your meals but you will also be filling your body with goodness and starving candida all at the same time. I wish you good health!

Notes about Ingredients

Flour

The wheat flour you use *must* be 100 per cent wholewheat (or wholemeal). Even 85 per cent will not do. Granary flour is no good because it is either white flour or part white and part wholemeal with added malt and grains. White flour has been refined, which means that it has been stripped of its nutrients and had various things added, like bleach and preservatives. This all has adverse effects on the body, including creating an imbalance of minerals and an increase of sugar in the blood. Most manufacturers who produce wholewheat flour supply it as either plain or self-raising and, although self-raising wholewheat flour is easier to use, its raising agent contains salt in the form of bicarbonate of soda (sodium bicarbonate) so it is best, if possible, to use plain wholewheat flour and add a salt-free raising agent *(see following point)*.

Raising Agents

Most shop-bought baking powder not only contains sodium bicarbonate, a form of salt, but also wheatflour, which is simply another name for refined white flour. A preferable alternative to sodium bicarbonate, in order to avoid the salt content, is potassium bicarbonate, which you might be able to buy from your local pharmacist or health-food store. As it is not always easily available, you might need to make a compromise and use sodium bicarbonate. However, by putting together your own raising agents – even if you have to use sodium bicarbonate instead of potassium bicarbonate – you are at least avoiding the refined flour content of commercial baking powders, and you will probably be avoiding something else which is rather more significant.

An essential part of baking powders is an acid ingredient to activate the bicarbonate. For this reason, in some recipes in this book you will find that yoghurt is included as well as bicarbonate, and this is because yoghurt contains lactic acid, providing the acid activator. But what can you use in recipes which contain no yoghurt, or if you cannot use yoghurt because you have a dairy intolerance? You have to find another form of acid.

In most bought baking powders, the acid activator is in the form of tartaric acid, or cream of tartar, and in the first edition of this book I recommended its use. However, I have since learned a thing or two about tartaric acid which means that I can no longer recommend it. For one thing, it is a highly toxic substance and, according to Dr William Shaw (*see Resources, page 281*), as little as 12 grams has caused human fatality (one gram being approximately the weight of a cigarette). The other major factor is that tartaric acid is a compound which is derived from yeast, and studies of children with autism and patients with fibromyalgia have found very high levels of tartaric acid in their urine, sometimes as much as 600 times above average. When these patients have been treated for yeast infection, the levels of tartaric acid have fallen significantly. Since one of the effects of tartaric acid is to interfere with energy production in the body's cells (which probably goes a long way to explain why candida sufferers so often have to struggle with fatigue), it is perhaps not such a good idea to have extra tartaric acid in our food.

So, coming back to our need for an efficient acid activator, a simple and effective alternative to tartaric acid or yoghurt is lemon juice. You will therefore find in each recipe requiring a raising agent a combination of potassium (or sodium) bicarbonate either with yoghurt or with lemon juice, mixed in at an appropriate stage. If that doesn't make your baking rise, I'll eat my hat!

Oil

Whichever type of oil you buy, make sure it is in a cold-pressed, unrefined form. Olive oil should be labelled *Extra Virgin*. Oils which are not cold-pressed provide a very serious health risk because they generate dangerous molecules called free radicals, which cause a chain-reaction of damaged cells in the body leading to health problems ranging from allergy to heart disease and even cancer.

For baking: Use cold-pressed, unrefined sunflower, safflower, linseed (flax) or olive oils or unsalted butter or unhydrogenated margarine.

For roasting or frying (for instance, softening onions): Use only extra virgin olive oil or unsalted butter. In fact, don't fry at all if you can grill or bake instead, and onions will soften very well in a little juice from a tin of tomatoes. You can roast a chicken or even a shoulder of lamb in a tin with a very little water in the bottom – no added fat at all.

For salad dressings: Cold-pressed, unrefined sunflower, safflower or linseed oils are actually more beneficial than olive oil when taken cold.

Eggs

Always buy free-range eggs; you may use either medium or large in recipes, making up the quantity of fluid with soya milk, if necessary. If you need to avoid eggs, or wish to reduce them, use soya milk instead in recipes which require binding (or a mixture of 2 tbsp of soya flour and a little water), and tofu in quiches and flans.

Soya Milk

Always check the packet carefully to make sure it contains no sugar, salt or apple juice. Try different makes to find one you really like – the taste can vary tremendously. If you really don't like soya milk, or have an intolerance to it, or simply want to increase variety (which is always a good idea), try rice milk, either plain or vanilla flavoured. This is another milk-substitute and it is made from organic whole-grain rice. It hadn't appeared when the first edition of this book was published, but it has become an extremely useful ingredient of the anti-candida diet so I gladly include it in this new edition.

Seasoning

Salt: You need to keep salt to an absolute minimum because it stimulates the adrenals which means that you end up with extra sugar in your blood. However, so many useful products contain it (for instance, cans of tomatoes and chickpeas) that it is virtually impossible to avoid it completely. Never add it to your cooking and learn to add less at table. Until your taste buds can cope with no added salt at all, use a product called 'Lo-Salt'; it tastes just as good but is in fact mostly potassium. If you have difficulty getting used to the flavour of some of the wholefoods, just a pinch of 'Lo-Salt' can make all the difference because it will seem more like the flavours you are used to. Once the level of zinc has been raised in your body, you will find that all foods have more flavour than you ever knew, and salt will not be necessary.

The only exception to the no-salt rule might be when someone is in a hot, humid climate causing excess perspiration and having a low intake of fresh vegetables.

Pepper: To avoid mould in pepper pots, it is best to use freshly-ground black peppercorns.

Carob

Carob powder is a healthy alternative to chocolate or cocoa powder, being free of natural stimulants, so it makes a good occasional treat for children. However, it has a natural sweetness which your candida will quite enjoy, so I suggest you play safe and use it only occasionally – in fact, I think grown-ups should mostly manage without it.

Organic Foods

It is tremendously encouraging that organically-produced food is now so readily available, not only in health-food stores but in the main supermarkets as well. Some butchers make a point of selling organically-reared meat, and its quality makes the extra cost very worthwhile, as does the flavour of organic vegetables. The main advantage is that it reduces the toxic load which enters your body. However, if you cannot afford organic food, still eat plenty of vegetables for their high fibre and vitamin and mineral content, and your supplement programme will help your body to deal with pollution from pesticides, etc. My advice is to enjoy organic food if you can, but don't get too stressed about it if you cannot.

Ten Further Tips

1) **Thickening.** You can experiment with different flours to thicken sauces and gravies – wholewheat flour, oatflour (fine oatmeal), whole rice flour, arrowroot or fine maize meal, which is the unrefined form of cornflour (cornstarch) and particularly useful. If you cook more vegetables than are needed, you can purée them to thicken your sauce or gravy (made from meat and/or vegetable juices) without needing flour.

2) **Adapting.** You can use any recipe from any book simply by exchanging white flour for wholemeal flour, milk for soya milk, vinegar for lemon juice, etc., etc.

3) **Lemon juice.** If you heat the lemon briefly in the microwave, you will find it squeezes much more easily and even produces more juice.

4) **Children.** Growing children need calcium, so you should make sure they have plenty of natural yoghurt, cottage cheese, green leafy vegetables and ground seeds, especially sesame. Your nutritionist will advise you on quantities of calcium and magnesium to supplement, depending on age and other factors. Crush the tablets and add to yoghurt, porridge or other food. This is particularly important if your child has a dairy intolerance. Children cope very well with the anti-candida diet if they understand the reason for it and are encouraged by a helpful attitude from parents and family who are prepared to join them on it. They can be far more strong-minded than grown-ups and many a child has happily taken his box of special food to a birthday party.

5) **Cheese for the family.** If you are serving a pasta meal and you are the only one on the anti-candida diet, serve some grated cheese separately. An alternative topping which is generally popular is a mixture of dry-roasted sunflower and sesame seeds, sprinkled on, ground or whole.

6) **Canned tomatoes.** These are a great time-saver, as long as you use them in moderation because they don't have all the benefits of fresh tomatoes. Make sure they have no added citric acid; these are not too easy to find, but they are available.

7) **Canned beans.** Not the ones with 57 varieties! Many supermarkets sell different types of beans and pulses (haricot, butterbeans, flageolet, kidney, black eye, chickpeas, lentils) ready-cooked in salted water. These save a great deal of time and

energy, but be sure to rinse them *very* well to remove as much salt as possible. Some cans also contain sugar, and these of course should be avoided like the plague! Rinsing well also removes the floury substance which clings to beans, and which is largely responsible for causing problems of intestinal gas.

8) **Cook double quantities.** Freeze half and save time and energy.

9) **Mixing liquid into recipes.** The amount of liquid indicated in any recipe should only ever be regarded as approximate. Different grains and flours absorb at different rates, whether you are adding water, soya milk or rice milk. Since making a mixture too stiff or too sloppy can ruin the end results, it is wise to add in the liquid ingredients just one tablespoonful at a time. That way you keep careful control over the consistency. Don't worry if you don't need all the fluid – or if you have to add a little more.

10) **Don't mix measurements.** Use *either* pounds and ounces *or else* kilos and grams (cup measurements are also given for American readers). Both are given in the recipes but they are *not* interchangeable, so if you try to mix them the recipe won't work properly. Please note that 'tsp' means a 5ml teaspoon, and 'tbsp' means a tablespoon which will hold three teaspoonsful. These measures should always be level unless the recipe states 'heaped'.

MOST OF THE FOLLOWING RECIPES ALLOW FOR FOUR SERVINGS UNLESS OTHERWISE STATED.

ENJOY THE END RESULTS!!

part two:

Recipes

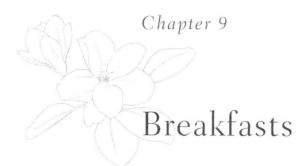

Chapter 9

Breakfasts

reakfast is for many people the biggest problem of the day, and yet it is also the most important meal. Many 'yeasties' suffer from symptoms associated with low blood sugar which, apart from anything else, will add to their general exhaustion and lack of energy. Breakfast, preferably containing protein, is a most important part of the programme to regulate low blood sugar. Even without this added complication, breakfast is vitally important. All my early knowledge of nutrition came from the books of Adelle Davis, who insisted we should 'Breakfast like a king, lunch like a prince and dine like a pauper!' So here are some ideas for breakfasts fit for a king.

Cereals

You can choose between shredded wheat, puffed wheat or whole puffed rice, all of which should be stocked by most well-known supermarkets. Another alternative is muesli base, for which you will need to find a wholefood shop. These cereals can be served with natural low-fat yoghurt or soya milk to provide protein, or with rice milk. Goat's milk contains nearly the same amount of lactose as cow's milk, so it is best avoided for the time being. Some folk like to soften their cereal overnight in a little filtered water – especially if it's muesli base – and then serve it with yoghurt. The pre-soaking makes it more easily digestible. If you like hot milk on your cereal, you could try flavouring some heated soya milk with a few drops of real vanilla essence, then pour it on shredded wheat with some freshly-cracked hazelnuts.

* Muesli Base

Muesli base is simply made up of your own mix of cereal flakes. Alternatively, you can buy it direct from a health-food store, but be careful to check it contains no dried fruits or nuts. Try the following mixture:

450g/1lb/2 cups jumbo oats
350g/12oz/3 cups wheat flakes
350g/12oz/3 cups barley flakes
350g/12oz/3 cups rye flakes

Try throwing in a handful of any seeds you fancy – sunflower, sesame, pumpkin or lin-seeds. Keep it all in an airtight container.

** Crunchy Breakfast Cereal

You can also use muesli base to make a crunchy breakfast cereal.

350g/12oz/3 cups muesli base
50g/2oz/½ cup wheatgerm
50g/2oz/½ cup sunflower seeds
50g/2oz/½ cup sesame seeds
50g/2oz/½ cup desiccated coconut
4–5 tbsp extra virgin olive oil

Heat the oven to 350°F/180°C/Gas Mark 4. Mix together all the ingredients and spread on a large baking sheet. Bake for 45 minutes, stirring every 10–15 minutes. Tip into another flat dish to cool before storing in an airtight container. Serve with natural yoghurt, or with hot or cold soya milk to provide protein.

* Oatmeal Porridge: Microwave Version

It seems that porridge is a favourite of many, and if you have a microwave it is particularly easy to make.

WHEAT-FREE, SERVES 2

1 cup porridge oats
2 cups water or soya milk (or half-and-half)
Optional: pinch of Lo-Salt

Cook, uncovered, on full power for 1½–2 minutes, stirring halfway through cooking time. Serve with a little cold soya milk poured over, or with natural yoghurt stirred in.

My own favourite version of this is made with jumbo oats and soya milk, using level measures of each. This makes it really thick and creamy. Topped with a sprinkling of cinnamon, it's quite delicious.

It's almost as easy to make porridge in a saucepan, but you're left with a sticky pan to clean. Make sure you fill it with water as soon as you've poured the porridge.

* Oatmeal Porridge: Saucepan Version

WHEAT-FREE, SERVES 2

Ingredients as for Microwave Version (*above*). Heat in a saucepan, stirring all the time, and boil for one minute.

* Oatmeal Breakfast

WHEAT-FREE

An alternative to porridge oats is coarse oatmeal. You can make breakfast for four very quickly by preparing it the night before.

150g/5oz/1 cup coarse oatmeal
1.2 litres/2 pints/5 cups boiling water
Optional: cinnamon or freshly-grated nutmeg

Pour the boiling water over the oatmeal in a saucepan and leave overnight. In the morning, bring to the boil, stirring, then reduce heat and simmer for 10 minutes until all the water is absorbed. Serve with natural yoghurt or with hot or cold soya milk or rice milk. Sprinkle with spice if desired.

Rice and Millet

An alternative to oat breakfasts is to use whole rice flakes. This enables you to rotate the grains, which is a good idea, and is also very useful on a gluten-free regime. For other gluten-free breakfasts you can use whole rice and millet. They are easily prepared in a slow-cooker, but to save making it every night you can keep spare portions in the refrigerator and reheat next morning, stirring well with some extra soya milk (use saucepan or microwave).

* Creamy Rice Breakfast

GLUTEN-FREE

1 mug whole rice
4 mugs soya milk
Optional: cinnamon or freshly-grated nutmeg

Cook overnight in a slow-cooker (8–9 hours). Stir well.

* Creamy Millet

GLUTEN-FREE

1 mug whole millet
4 mugs soya milk
Optional: cinnamon or freshly-grated nutmeg

Cook overnight in a slow-cooker (8 hours). It tends to stick to the bottom, so stir well before serving.

Sago and Tapioca

Notable but unfortunate omissions in the first edition of this book were sago and tapioca, both of which are quite acceptable for the anti-candida diet. They seem to be not nearly so widely used as they were in my childhood; maybe memories of school dinners has led to a slump in sales among adults! Who could ever forget the frogspawn-like version of chocolate tapioca pudding? However, it is worth putting such memories behind you and seeing what you can do with these useful foods.

What exactly are they? Sago is a starch derived from the powdered pith of the sago palm tree. Tapioca is also a starch, derived from the roots of a plant called cassava. Since neither of them are grains, it means that they are extremely useful for a gluten-free diet and in most cases also for a diet which is free of all grains, although some people with a high intolerance to starchy foods should try them with caution.

---

* Sago or Tapioca Breakfast

GLUTEN-FREE, GRAIN-FREE, SERVES 1

The following breakfast recipe could equally well be used as a dessert.

75g/3oz/½ cup sago or tapioca
Good sprinkling of mixed spice
150–425ml/¼–¾ pint/⅔–2 cups soya milk

Microwave: Put tapioca or sago into a large microwave bowl and sprinkle with mixed spice. Add 150ml/¼ pint/⅔ cup of soya milk, stir and microwave on High for 5 minutes (based on 800W microwave). Stir again, add more milk and cook for another 5 minutes on High. Stir again. (It will be thick by now.) Put into a cereal bowl and add more cold soya milk.

Conventional oven: Allow 40g/1½oz sago or tapioca to 600ml/1 pint/2½ cups soya milk. Preheat oven to 300°F/150°C/Gas Mark 2. Pour mixture into a greased pie dish and cook slowly for 2 hours or longer. Make the previous evening and then reheat in a saucepan for breakfast, stirring well.

Yoghurt

The easiest protein breakfast of all is a bowl of low-fat natural yoghurt. You will find more about yoghurt in Chapter 28, 'Desserts', where I explain the different types available and how to make your own. For now, let's consider it as an easy-to-digest, good quality protein breakfast dish, on its own or dressed up a little as in the following recipe.

Yoghurt Surprise

SERVES 1 OR 2

Small tub natural yoghurt
1 tbsp pumpkin seeds
1 tbsp sunflower seeds
1 tbsp linseeds
1 tbsp wheatgerm
Optional: 1 tbsp lecithin granules
Optional: 2 tbsp whole puffed rice

Mix together all the ingredients. Greek yoghurt may be used, but try to find the low-fat variety, or make your own as described on page 68.

Toast or Crackers and Spreads

Yoghurt soda bread (*see Chapter 10*) can be eaten sliced as it is or toasted, and is delicious with unhydrogenated margarine, cottage cheese or seedy butter (*see overleaf*). Alternatives to soda bread are bought rice cakes and crispbreads made from wholewheat or rye, or any others you can find which are made from a whole grain and free of additives as well as yeast.

* Seedy Butter

GLUTEN-FREE

Seedy butter must be one of the most easy, tasty and nutritious spreads ever invented, but you do need a grinder to make it *(see page 105)*.

* Toast and Seedy Butter

Slice some wholemeal, yeast-free soda bread and spread it with seedy butter. Cover with sliced tomatoes and pop under a hot grill for 1 minute.

Eggs

Free-range eggs make an excellent high-protein breakfast. Have them boiled, poached or scrambled, but never fried. Because of their fat content, keep your egg intake to about five per week – and that includes those you use in baking. (Try using 2 tbsp of soya flour with a little water instead of an egg in baking recipes.)

* Scrambled Eggs: Microwave Version

GLUTEN-FREE, SERVES 1 OR 2

2 free-range eggs
2 tbsp soya milk
Freshly ground black pepper

Beat ingredients in a jug or bowl, and cook uncovered for about 2–2½ minutes, stirring every half-minute.

* Scrambled Eggs: Saucepan Version

Ingredients as for Microwave Version except that you need to add a knob of unsalted butter. Melt the butter in a saucepan and let it coat the bottom and sides before you add the mixture. Beat eggs, soya milk and seasoning in a bowl and pour into the coated saucepan. Cook over a low heat, stirring all the time, until set and creamy. Serve on toasted soda bread or eat with rice cakes and unhydrogenated margarine.

Tofu

Tofu is a curd made from soya beans and you will learn a little more about how to use it on pages 217–18. It makes a good alternative to eggs in many recipes.

* Scrambled Tofu

SERVES 1 OR 2

½ packet (about 5oz/150g) tofu
1 tomato, chopped
Freshly ground black pepper
Optional: pinch of Lo-salt
Toasted wholemeal yeast-free soda bread

Mash tofu with the tomato and add seasoning. Spread over toast and grill for 2–3 minutes. Couldn't be easier!.

Other Breakfast Ideas

Other ways of having protein at breakfast may seem a little more unusual but can be very enjoyable, and they certainly give you a good start to the day. For instance, there is no reason why you shouldn't have fish or chicken for breakfast, and for someone with low blood sugar this is an excellent idea. Again, a microwave makes it easy to cook a cod portion with tomatoes, or a chicken drumstick, but even without a microwave it takes very little time to poach a piece of fish in a pan of boiling water, and with a little fore-thought you could have some pre-cooked drumsticks in the refrigerator. Canned tuna or pink salmon with tomatoes and cucumber gives a good combination of protein and complex carbohydrate, as well as essential fatty acids.

With so many possibilities to choose from, you will probably find that breakfast is much more interesting than it ever was before you started the anti-candida diet. I highly recommend pease pudding grilled with tomatoes (*see page 268*).

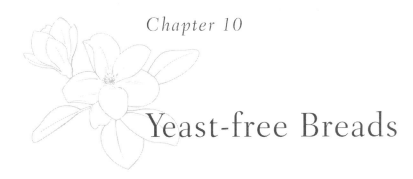

Yeast-free Breads

Although yeast-free bread is extremely quick and easy to make, I have put it into the ** category because it does entail some mixing. If you are just 'SURVIVING' at the moment, you will probably need to ask friends or relations to make you a batch of bread to put in the freezer, and some helpful bakers' shops and delicatessens will actually make up a batch to your own recipe. It's worth enquiring.

It is perfectly possible to live on the anti-candida diet without eating bread, because so many other 'fillers' are available in the shops, from rice cakes (which look like ceiling tiles but taste delicious!), to whole rye crispbread (take care to avoid those with malt in), wholewheat crackers and oat cakes (though again read the label because many of these also contain malt).

The bread recipes which follow are so easy and so delicious that, if you're not careful, you will find yourself putting on weight! Perhaps the most useful time to have some bread available is at Sunday teatime, which for many is traditionally a time for starchy foods and so causes problems on the anti-candida diet. The chapters on 'Spreads and Dips', 'Biscuits', and 'Cakes and Scones' will help here, also.

Before you go on to use the recipes, I suggest that you look back to page 56 where I discussed the various types of flour available and the best ones to use, also the different types of fat and oil and the pros and cons of raising agents.

72

** Yoghurt Soda Bread

This basic bread recipe is a firm favourite, and many of my clients have produced variations on the theme.

450g/1lb/3¼ cups wholewheat plain flour
2 tsp potassium (or sodium) bicarbonate
300ml/½ pint/1⅓ cups natural yoghurt
150ml/¼ pint/⅔ cup warm filtered water

This will make two small loaves or one large one. If you want to make a batch for the freezer, a 1.5kg/3½lb bag of flour and a 1-litre/1¾-pint tub of yoghurt (with 6 tsp bicarbonate and ½ litre/¾ pint warm water) makes six small loaves. Preheat the oven to 400°F/200°C/Gas Mark 6. Sift the flour and mix in the raising agent, then stir in the yoghurt and warm water. Mix together well then coat the mixture with more flour and liberally flour your working surface. No kneading is necessary. If making small loaves, divide into two and make into fairly flat, oval shapes. Cut a cross on the top. Place on a floured tray and bake for 30 minutes, then turn oven down to 350°F/180°C/Gas Mark 4 for another 20 minutes. To test if it's ready, tap the bottom of the loaf and it should sound hollow. Leave to cool on a wire rack. Six loaves in the oven might require a little more baking time.

** Seedy Yoghurt Soda Bread

Make the mixture as for Plain Yoghurt Soda Bread and throw in a handful of sunflower seeds and a handful of pumpkin seeds. This makes it rather like a granary loaf.

** Oaty Yoghurt Soda Bread

Make the mixture as for Plain Yoghurt Soda Bread except that you take out 2 tablespoons of flour from the original weight and replace it with coarse oatmeal. Instead of coating the dough with flour, coat it with more oatmeal. Top with poppy seeds and you'll be amazed at how professional it looks!

** Soya Milk Loaf

This recipe is slightly different, using soya milk instead of yoghurt.

450g/1lb/3¼ cups wholewheat flour
1 tsp potassium (or sodium) bicarbonate
2 tsp fresh lemon juice
1 tbsp extra virgin olive oil
Soya milk to mix (or 2 heaped tbsp soya flour with 350ml/12fl oz/1½ cups water)
Optional: poppy seeds to decorate

Preheat oven to 400°F/200°C/Gas Mark 6. Mix raising agent with flour, stir in the lemon juice, then rub in the oil. Add sufficient soya milk to make a soft dough, probably just over 300ml/½ pint. Coat well with flour, shape into a round and cut a deep cross on the top. Sprinkle with poppy seeds if using. Place on a baking tray and bake for 30 minutes. Cool on a wire rack.

   To microwave, place on microwave dish and cook on High for 6½ minutes (600w).

** Coconut Loaf

A variation on the Soya Milk Loaf is made with the following ingredients in place of the 450g/1lb/3¼ cups wholewheat flour.

350g/12oz/2½ cups wholewheat flour
125g/4oz/⅔ cup fine oatmeal
50g/2oz/½ cup desiccated coconut

Mix in the remaining ingredients and bake as for Soya Milk Loaf.

Bread Rolls and Tin Loaves

Any of the bread mixtures may be used to make small rolls. Cook for 20 minutes at 400°F/200°C/Gas Mark 6 and then 10 minutes at 350°F/180°C/Gas Mark 4. These are lovely eaten warm with soup if your digestion is up to it!

Tin-shaped loaves are easier to slice for toast and sandwiches than oval ones, and for these the mixture needs to be even more moist and sticky. Put the dough into a greased 1kg/2lb tin, or two ½kg/1lb tins, and smooth the top with a wooden spoon. Bake the large loaf for 20 minutes at 400°F/200°C/Gas Mark 6 followed by 30 minutes at 350°F/180°C/Gas Mark 4, and the small loaves need just slightly less cooking time at the lower heat.

** Tea Bread

The addition of an egg gives bread a more cake-like texture.

225g/8oz/1½ cups plain wholewheat flour
1 tsp potassium (or sodium) bicarbonate
2 tsp fresh lemon juice
1 tbsp extra virgin olive oil
1 free-range egg
150ml/¼ pint/⅔ cup soya milk (or rice milk)
Sesame seeds for topping

Preheat oven to 375°F/190°C/Gas Mark 5. Sift and mix the flour and bicarbonate powder. Stir in the lemon juice and oil. Beat the egg and soya milk together and add to mixture. Mix to a stiff batter and put into a greased ½ kg/1lb loaf tin. Bake for 45 minutes. It's easy to double the mixture and make two at a time, one to freeze.

Wheat-free Breads

The next recipes use grains other than wheat, so are useful if you suffer from wheat intolerance, and the final ideas for corn bread are suitable for a gluten-free diet (*see also pages 76–7*).

* Easy Oat Bread 1

WHEAT-FREE

300g/10oz/1¾ cups fine oatmeal
1 tsp potassium (or sodium) bicarbonate
1 tbsp natural yoghurt
Filtered water to mix

Sift oatmeal and bicarbonate powder and add yoghurt and water till you have a sloppy batter. (The oatmeal absorbs a lot of water.) Use a ½kg/1lb loaf-tin brushed with oil, pour in the batter and bake at 350°F/180°C/Gas Mark 4 until risen (about 35–40 minutes).

* Oat Bread 2

WHEAT-FREE

400g/15oz/2½ cups oats
75g/3oz/½ cup soya flour
Handful sunflower seeds
3 tbsp extra virgin olive oil
Hot filtered water to mix

Preheat oven to 375°F/190°C/Gas Mark 5. Mix together the oats, soya flour and sunflower seeds. Stir in the oil and mix with hot water to make a dough consistency. Shape into a ball, using oats to coat the dough. Cut a cross on top, place on a baking tray and bake for 30–40 minutes. Check when done by tapping the bottom for a hollow sound. Cool on a wire rack.

** Corn Bread

GLUTEN-FREE

This recipe has a nice 'cakey' texture but does tend to become dry after a couple of days, so it needs eating quickly unless you use it for toast, which is delicious!

125g/4oz/1 cup fine maize meal
125g/4oz/1 cup soya flour
60g/2oz/½ cup whole (brown) rice flour
2 tsp potassium (or sodium) bicarbonate
1 cup soya milk
1 free-range egg (or slightly more soya milk)
4 tsp fresh lemon juice

Preheat oven to 375°F/190°C/Gas Mark 5. Mix the dry ingredients. Beat egg (if using) and soya milk together and add to the mixture together with lemon juice. Place in a greased loaf tin and bake for about 30 minutes. Turn out and cool on a wire rack. You may think this recipe has a rather strong taste of soya flour when first cooked, but in fact that mellows after a while. It can be avoided by exchanging the quantities of rice flour and soya flour, i.e. 1 cup brown rice flour, ½ cup soya flour.

---

* Moist Corn Bread

GLUTEN-FREE

If you prefer a loaf which keeps moist longer, try this recipe.

125g/4oz/1 cup fine maize meal
60g/2oz/½ cup soya flour
125g/4oz/1 cup whole (brown) rice flour
1 tsp potassium (or sodium) bicarbonate
1½ tbsp extra virgin olive oil
2 tsp fresh lemon juice
1–2 cups soya milk (or rice milk)

Preheat oven to 400°F/200°C/Gas Mark 6. Mix dry ingredients and stir in the oil and lemon juice. Add sufficient soya milk to obtain a dropping consistency. Place in a greased loaf tin and bake for 30 minutes. Cool on a wire rack.

** Carrot Bread

GLUTEN-FREE

150g/6oz/1¼ cups brown rice flour
2 free-range eggs, beaten
2 cups grated carrot (and/or parsnip)
¾ cup extra virgin olive oil
2 tsp potassium (or sodium) bicarbonate
2 tbsp natural yoghurt
½ tsp freshly grated nutmeg
½ tsp ground cinnamon
1–2 tsp vanilla essence, according to taste
1–2 tbsp seeds from among sesame, linseed (flax-seed), sunflower, as preferred

Preheat oven to 325°/170°/Gas Mark 3. Mix all ingredients together (in a food processor if you have one) and spoon into a 500g/1lb greased loaf-tin. Bake for 1 hour. This client says that brown rice flour tastes especially good when it has been freshly ground at home!

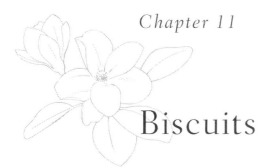

Chapter 11

Biscuits

So often, people are afraid they will have to starve on the anti-candida diet and cannot imagine life without biscuits. If you feel like this, the good news for you is that you don't have to live without biscuits! It is quite possible to come up with crunchy cookies made with the allowed ingredients. Once you have lost your sweet tooth (and you will when you no longer encourage it, because you weren't born with it), you will appreciate the flavours of other ingredients so much more, and find these sugar-free biscuits just as moreish as you used to find the ones in a packet. Biscuits make good additions to packed lunches, and are also very useful for children. Oatcakes with spreads make a good filler, providing an alternative to bread.

* Oatcakes 1

WHEAT-FREE

150g/5oz/1 scant cup medium oatmeal
1 tsp unsalted butter
125ml/4fl oz/½ cup boiling filtered water

Preheat oven to 350°F/180°C/Gas Mark 4. Put oatmeal into a bowl. Put butter into a heatproof jug and pour the boiling water onto it. When butter has melted, pour liquid onto the oatmeal and mix well. Leave for a few minutes till oatmeal swells and becomes workable. Turn onto a well-floured board and divide into two balls. Roll each ball into a small round and cut across it four times to make eight wedges. Roll each wedge very thinly. Place on baking sheet and bake for about 30 minutes. Wedges will be slightly curved and lightly golden.

** Oatcakes 2

225g/8oz/1⅓ cups oatmeal
125g/4oz/1 cup plain wholemeal flour
1 tsp potassium (or sodium) bicarbonate
75g/3oz/⅓ cup unsalted butter
2 tsp fresh lemon juice
6 tbsp filtered water (approximately)

Preheat oven to 350°F/180°C/Gas Mark 4. Mix dry ingredients, rub in the butter then stir in the lemon juice and water to make a stiff dough. Knead briefly on a floured surface and roll out thinly. Cut rounds with the top of a small glass or a pastry-cutter. Cover baking sheet with greaseproof paper brushed with melted butter or olive oil. Bake for 35 minutes. Cool on a wire rack.

** Coconut Biscuits

MAY BE WHEAT-FREE

50g/2oz/½ cup desiccated coconut
125g/4oz/1 cup plain wholemeal flour
½ tsp potassium (or sodium) bicarbonate
50g/2oz/¼ cup unsalted butter (or 2 tbsp extra virgin olive oil)
1 tsp fresh lemon juice
1 free-range egg

Variations: instead of wholemeal flour, use 25g/1oz brown rice flour, 40g/1½oz/⅓ cup fine maize meal and 40g/1½oz/⅓ cup barley flour.

Preheat oven to 350°F/180°/Gas Mark 4. Mix dry ingredients, rub in butter or oil then add beaten egg and lemon juice (or place all ingredients together in a food processor). Make one rounded teaspoonful into a ball and press flat with your hands. Place on a baking tray which has been covered with greaseproof paper and brushed with melted butter or olive oil. Continue to make biscuits in this way until all the dough has been used up. Bake for 20 minutes. Leave to cool on tray.

** Ginger Cookies

150g/5oz/1 cup plain wholemeal flour
½ tsp potassium (or sodium) bicarbonate
25g/1oz oatmeal
2 tsp ground ginger
1 tsp ground coriander
50g/2oz/¼ cup unsalted butter
1 free-range egg
4 tsp soya milk (or rice milk)
1 tsp fresh lemon juice

Preheat oven to 350°F/180°C/Gas Mark 4. Mix dry ingredients and rub in butter. Lightly beat egg with soya milk and lemon juice, add to dry ingredients and mix to a soft dough. Knead on floured surface and roll thinly. Cut rounds with top of small glass or pastry cutter. Place on a lined baking try as above, and bake for 30 minutes. Cool on a wire rack.

** Sesame Cookies

175g/6oz/1¼ cups plain wholemeal flour
25g/1oz oatmeal
½ tsp potassium (or sodium) bicarbonate
75g/3oz/⅓ cup unsalted butter
50g/2oz/½ cup sesame seeds
4 tbsp soya milk (or rice milk)
1 tsp fresh lemon juice

Preheat oven to 350°F/180°C/Gas Mark 4. Mix flour, oatmeal and bicarbonate powder, rub in butter and add sesame seeds. Stir in soya milk and lemon juice, mixing to a firm dough. Roll out thinly on floured surface, cut rounds with top of small glass or pastry-cutter, place on lined baking tray as above. Bake for 35 minutes. Cool on wire rack.

** Pastry Cookies

Make pastry to chosen recipe (*see pages 99–102*). Preheat oven to 350°F/180°C/Gas Mark 4. To approximately 225g/8oz pastry (made up of whichever flours you are using), add any of the following ingredients to make a variety of cookies, then proceed as follows:

Roll out thinly on floured surface, cut into rounds and place on lined baking tray, as above. Bake for 30 minutes. Cool on a wire rack.

** Carob Cookies

Replace 2 tbsp flour with 2 tbsp carob powder.

** Vanilla Cookies

Add 1–2 tsp of natural vanilla essence to pastry mix.

** Almond Cookies

Add 1–2 tsp of natural almond essence to pastry mix.

** Nut Cookies

Add 50g/2oz/½ cup chopped freshly cracked nuts to pastry mix.

** Seedy Cookies

Add 2 tbsp sunflower or sesame seeds to pastry mix.

Carob Biscuits

The following biscuit recipes use carob, which makes a special treat for children, but please read my comments on page 58.

** Carob Biscuits

GLUTEN-FREE

25g/1oz whole rice flour
50g/2oz/⅓ cup soya flour
75g/3oz/½ cup fine maize meal (unrefined cornflour/cornstarch)
50g/2oz/½ cup carob powder
2 tbsp extra virgin olive oil
Juice of 2 lemons made up to 50ml/2fl oz with filtered water
70ml/2½ fl oz/¼ cup natural yoghurt (or 2 free-range eggs, beaten)

Preheat oven to 375°F/190°C/Gas Mark 5. Mix dry ingredients, add the oil and rub to breadcrumb consistency. Add liquid and yoghurt or eggs, mixing well to form a soft dough. Flatten to 12mm/½-inch thickness and cut into shapes. Place on lined baking tray and bake for 15–20 minutes.

** Carob Cookies

175g/6oz/1¼ cups plain wholemeal flour
50g/2oz/⅓ cup oatmeal
2 tbsp carob powder
½ tsp potassium (or sodium) bicarbonate

75g/3oz/⅓ cup unsalted butter
4 tbsp soya milk (or rice milk)
1 tsp fresh lemon juice

Preheat oven to 350°F/180°/Gas Mark 4. Mix dry ingredients and rub in butter. Add soya milk and lemon juice, mixing to a firm dough. Roll to 12mm/½-inch thickness, cut into rounds or shapes and bake on a lined baking tray for 35 minutes. Cool on a wire rack.

---

* Carob Chip Cookies

125g/4oz/½ cup unsalted butter (or unhydrogenated margarine)
1 free-range egg
150g/5oz/1 cup plain wholemeal flour
½ bar carob confection bar (dairy-free, sugar-free), chopped

Preheat oven to 350°F/180°C/Gas Mark 4. Beat fat and egg. Add flour and pieces of carob bar. Mix and form into balls. Place on greased baking tray and bake for 20 minutes. If possible, eat the same day, otherwise freeze the unbaked mixture and bake a small amount at a time.

---

* Carob and Coconut Shortbread

125g/4oz/½ cup unsalted butter
175g/6oz/1¼ cups plain wholewheat flour
25g/1oz/¼ cup carob powder
25g/1oz/⅓ cup desiccated coconut

Preheat oven to 350°F/180°C/Gas Mark 4. Rub all ingredients together. Press into shallow, lightly greased and floured tin and bake for 25 minutes.

Variations: add cinnamon; vary carob content according to taste; use gluten-free flours.

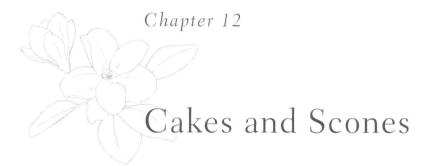

Chapter 12

Cakes and Scones

I f you have a food processor, any of the following recipes would obviously be easier to make and could even be given a * rating.

** (*) Basic Carrot Cake 1

1 free-range egg
4 tbsp unsalted butter
2 cups grated carrot
250g/8oz/1½ cups plain wholemeal flour
1 tsp potassium (or sodium) bicarbonate
½ tsp ground cinnamon
2 tsp fresh lemon juice
Soya milk (or rice milk), to mix

Preheat oven to 325°F/160°C/Gas Mark 3. Beat together the egg and butter then fold in the grated carrot. Sift together the dry ingredients and mix in well. Add lemon juice and soya or rice milk till mixture just drops off the spoon. Pour into a loaf tin which has been brushed with olive oil or melted butter and bake for 1 hour. Allow to stand a little, then turn out carefully onto a wire rack to cool.

Variations

** (*) Nutty Carrot Cake

Add a few nuts, freshly cracked and chopped.

** (*) Beany Carrot Cake

Add 2 tbsp of any variety of cooked or canned beans *(see page 166)*.

** (*)Carrot and Parsnip Cake

Replace one cup of grated carrot with one cup of grated parsnip.

** (*) Basic Carrot Cake 2

150g/5oz/1 cup plain wholemeal flour
1 tsp potassium (or sodium) bicarbonate
1 tsp ground cinnamon
1 tsp ground nutmeg
125g/4oz/½ cup unsalted butter (or 4 tbsp unrefined sunflower oil)
2 free-range eggs
50g/2oz/⅓ cup finely grated carrot
2 tsp fresh lemon juice

Preheat oven to 400°F/200°C/Gas Mark 6. Sift and mix flour, bicarbonate powder, cinnamon and nutmeg. Cream the butter and beat in the eggs one at a time, using a spoonful of flour to mix with each one. Add the grated carrot and lemon juice then the rest of the flour mixture. Bake for 25 minutes in a sandwich tin lined with oiled greaseproof paper.

Erica White's Beat Candida Cookbook

** (*) Carrot and Lemon Cake

150g/5oz/1 cup plain wholemeal flour
2 tsp potassium (or sodium) bicarbonate
125g/4oz/1 scant cup brown rice flour
125g/4oz/½ cup unsalted butter
2 free-range eggs
1 organic lemon, grated rind and juice
2 medium carrots, finely grated

Variations: instead of 125g/4oz/1 scant cup rice flour, try half rice flour and half desiccated coconut, or replace 3 tbsp rice flour with 3 tbsp carob powder.

Preheat oven to 350°F/180°C/Gas Mark 4. Sift dry ingredients. Add remainder and beat until smooth. Turn into lined cake tin and bake for 40–50 minutes. Allow to stand for a few minutes before turning out onto a wire rack to cool.

** Lemon Sesame Cake

125g/4oz/½ cup unsalted butter
2 free-range eggs
225g/8oz/1½ cups plain wholemeal flour
2 tsp potassium (or sodium) bicarbonate
150g/5oz natural yoghurt
2 tbsp sesame seeds
1 large organic lemon, freshly grated rind and juice

Preheat oven to 325°F/160°C/Gas Mark 3. Cream together the butter and eggs. Sift flour and bicarbonate powder and add to butter and egg mixture. Fold in the yoghurt, and lastly fold in the sesame seeds and grated lemon rind and juice. Bake for about 1 hour until risen and firm to the touch. Cool on a wire rack.

** (*) Ginger Cake (or Ginger and Walnut)

125g/4oz/½ cup unsalted butter
2 free-range eggs
2½ tsp ground ginger
150g/5oz/1 cup plain wholemeal flour
1 tsp potassium (or sodium) bicarbonate
2 tsp fresh lemon juice
Optional: 50g/2oz freshly cracked chopped walnuts

Preheat oven to 400°F/200°C/Gas Mark 6. Cream the butter and eggs then sift the ginger with the flour and bicarbonate powder and add to mixture in the bowl. Add lemon juice, then the chopped walnuts if using, saving some pieces for the top. Bake in a lined sandwich tin for 20 minutes.

** (*) Carob Cake

225g/8oz/1½ cups plain wholemeal flour
1½ tsp potassium (or sodium) bicarbonate
3 tbsp carob powder
125g/4oz/1½ cups oats
225g/8oz/1 cup unsalted butter
150ml/¼ pint/⅔ cup soya milk (or rice milk)
3 tsp fresh lemon juice
1–2 tsp natural vanilla essence

Preheat oven to 375°F/190°C/Gas Mark 5. Sift flour with bicarbonate and carob powder and add the oats. Melt butter and mix with soya milk, lemon juice and vanilla essence, then add to flour mixture, stirring. Bake in a lined tin for 45 minutes and leave in tin till quite cool.

** Celebration Carob Cake

This carob cake is best eaten the same day. Alternatively, make it in a loaf-tin, cut it in half and put half in the freezer.

2 large sweet potatoes
125g/4oz/½ cup unsalted butter (or unhydrogenated margarine)
2 large free-range eggs, beaten
225g/8oz/1½ cups plain wholemeal flour
1 tsp potassium (or sodium) bicarbonate
2 tbsp carob powder
1 tsp ground cinnamon
2 tsp fresh lemon juice
Some loosely chopped, freshly-cracked walnuts or almonds

Filling:
50g/2oz/½–¾ cup unsalted butter (or unhydrogenated margarine)
Carob powder to taste

Topping:
1 carob confection bar (dairy-free, sugar-free)

Preheat oven to 350°F/180°C/Gas Mark 4. Boil the sweet potatoes till soft. Meanwhile, mix butter or margarine with the beaten eggs. Add all dry ingredients and lemon juice. Mash the sweet potatoes when cold and add to mixture. Nuts may be mixed in or placed on top. Bake in a lined tin for about 1 hour, but check after 45 minutes. When cooked, leave to cool then slice through the middle. Spread with butter or margarine mixed with a little carob powder and replace top of cake. For an extra special cake, melt the carob bar in a bowl over a pan of boiling water, quickly spread over the top of the cake and leave to set.

** (*) Batter Cakes

4 heaped tbsp plain wholemeal flour
½ tsp potassium (or sodium) bicarbonate
1 free-range egg
1 tsp fresh lemon juice
1 cup soya milk (or rice milk)

Preheat oven to 400°F/200°C/Gas Mark 6. Sift flour and bicarbonate. Add egg to flour, then add lemon juice. Gradually add soya milk, beating all the time. Wipe round some muffin or fairy cake tins with buttered greaseproof paper and heat the tins for 2 minutes. Pour in batter and bake on top shelf for 25 minutes. Be sure you don't open the door too soon or they will sink! Serve with cottage cheese, which may be mixed with some natural vanilla essence, if you like.

Treats for Children

** Fairy Coconut Cakes

Fairy cake cases
2 free-range eggs
120ml/4fl oz/½ cup unrefined sunflower oil
4 tsp fresh lemon juice
2 carrots, finely grated
175g/6oz/1¼ cups plain wholemeal flour
2 tsp potassium (or sodium) bicarbonate
50g/2oz/⅔ cup desiccated coconut

Preheat oven to 350°F/180°C/Gas Mark 4. Put cake cases into hollows in bun tray. Mix eggs, oil, lemon juice and grated carrots, and in a separate bowl mix the flour, bicarbonate and coconut. Combine the two mixtures and stir until completely smooth. Put into cake cases and bake for 20–25 minutes, until cakes are firm in the centre and spring back when lightly pressed.

---

* Carob Crunchies

MAY BE GLUTEN-FREE

50g/2oz/⅓ cup carob confection bar (dairy-free, sugar-free), broken into squares
2 cups whole-grain puffed rice (or whole-grain wheatflakes or puffed wheat)
Optional: 2 tbsp desiccated coconut
Fairy cake cases

Melt carob bar in a bowl over a saucepan of boiling water. Tip in the other ingredients and mix thoroughly till cereals are covered. Put into fairy cake cases, and set in refrigerator.

Scones and Teacakes

The following cakes, scones and teacakes are enjoyable with a scraping of unsalted butter or unhydrogenated margarine or they may be used with any of your favourite spreads (*see pages 103–9*).

---

* Rye Slice

75g/3oz/½ cup wholewheat flour
75g/3oz/½ cup rye flour
75g/3oz/½ cup barley flour
75g/3oz/½ cup soya flour
115g/4oz/1 cup rye flakes
3 tsp mixed spice
3 tbsp extra virgin olive oil
Boiling filtered water to mix

Preheat oven to 375°F/190°C/Gas Mark 5. Combine flours, flakes and spice and rub or stir in the oil. Pour on boiling water slowly, mixing to form a dough. Place into an oiled loaf tin and bake for 30–40 minutes. Alternatively, put into a suitable container and cook in the microwave on High for 6 minutes (600W). Cool on a rack. Serve sliced.

** Oatmeal Cake

WHEAT-FREE

225g/8oz/1⅔ cups fine oatmeal
1½ tsp potassium (or sodium) bicarbonate
125g/4oz/½ cup unsalted butter (or unhydrogenated margarine)
2 tbsp natural yoghurt
2 large free-range eggs
Optional added flavours: 4 tsp mixed spice, or grated rind and juice of an organic lemon

Preheat oven to 350°F/180°C/Gas Mark 4. Sift dry ingredients. Make sure butter or margarine is very soft, then add to mixture along with yoghurt and eggs. Also at this stage add any additional flavourings, such as spice or lemon. Beat well. Add water if needed to obtain a sloppy batter which falls off the spoon very easily. For a thick cake, use a 15cm/6-inch tin; for a thin cake use an 18cm/7-inch tin, lined with lightly oiled grease-proof paper. Bake for 45 minutes.

** Wholemeal Scones 1

150g/6oz/1 cup plain wholemeal flour (or half oatmeal or rye flour)
60g/2oz/½ cup whole rice flour
2 tsp fine maize meal
1 tsp potassium (or sodium) bicarbonate
40g/1½oz unsalted butter (or 2 tbsp unrefined sunflower oil)
1 free-range egg (or 2 tbsp soya flour)
2 tsp fresh lemon juice
1 tbsp soya milk (or rice milk)
1 tbsp filtered water

Preheat oven to 425°F/220°C/Gas Mark 7. Mix dry ingredients and rub in the butter. Mix together egg (if using), lemon juice, soya milk and water and add to mixture. Roll out on floured surface to 2cm/¾-inch thickness, and cut into rounds with top of a small glass or pastry-cutter. Bake on a floured tray for 10–15 minutes. Cool on wire rack.

** Wholemeal Scones 2

225g/8oz/1½ cups plain wholemeal flour
1 tsp potassium (or sodium) bicarbonate
50g/2oz/¼ cup unsalted butter
1 free-range egg (or 2 tbsp soya flour)
2 tsp fresh lemon juice
Soya milk (or rice milk), to mix

Preheat oven to 425°F/220°C/Gas Mark 7. Sift flour and bicarbonate powder and rub in the butter. Beat the egg and mix in, then add lemon juice and sufficient soya milk to make a firm dough. Knead lightly on a floured surface and roll out to 12mm/½-inch thickness. Cut into rounds and bake on lined baking tray. Bake for 12–15 minutes. Cool on wire rack.

** Herb Scones

125g/4oz/1 scant cup plain wholemeal flour
125g/4oz/¾ cup medium oatmeal
2 tsp potassium (or sodium) bicarbonate
¾ tsp mixed dried herbs (or ¼ each of rosemary, sage, parsley)
25g/1oz unsalted butter (or 1 tbsp unrefined sunflower oil)
4 tsp fresh lemon juice
150ml/¼ pint/⅔ cup soya milk (or rice milk)

Preheat oven to 450°F/230°C/Gas Mark 8. Mix together dry ingredients and rub in butter. Mix in lemon juice and enough soya milk to make a soft dough, the wetter the better – only just manageable. Then dust well with flour and press or roll on a floured surface to 12mm/½-inch thickness, and cut into rounds. Transfer to greased baking tray and bake for 8–10 minutes till risen. Cool on wire rack.

** Yoghurt Scones

225g/8oz/1½ cups plain wholemeal flour
½ tsp potassium (or sodium) bicarbonate
50g/2oz/¼ cup unsalted butter
150g/5oz natural yoghurt
Soya milk (or yoghurt and water) for brushing
Sesame seeds for sprinkling

Preheat oven to 425°F/220°C/Gas Mark 7. Sift flour and bicarbonate powder, rub in butter, add yoghurt and mix to a soft dough. Knead lightly on floured surface and roll to 18mm/¾-inch thickness. Cut into rounds and place on a floured baking sheet. Brush with soya milk or mixture of yoghurt and water and sprinkle with sesame seeds. Bake for 12–15 minutes. Cool on wire rack.

** Oaty Scones

125g/4oz/1½ cups porridge oats
125g/4oz/1 scant cup plain wholemeal flour
1 tsp potassium (or sodium) bicarbonate
50g/2oz/¼ cup unsalted butter (or 2 tbsp unrefined sunflower oil)
2 tsp fresh lemon juice
4–5 tbsp soya milk (or rice milk)

Preheat oven to 400°F/200°C/Gas Mark 6. Mix together dry ingredients and rub in butter. Stir in lemon juice and sufficient soya milk to make a pliable dough. Knead gently on a floured surface and roll out to 12mm/½-inch thickness. Cut rounds and place on floured baking tray. Brush with soya milk and sprinkle with oats. Bake for 12–15 minutes till risen and golden. Serve warm, or cool on a wire rack.

Erica White's Beat Candida Cookbook

** Rock Cake Scones

350g/12oz/2½ cups plain wholemeal flour
2 tsp potassium (or sodium) bicarbonate
175g/6oz/¾ cup unsalted butter (or 6 tbsp sunflower oil)
2 free-range eggs
4 tsp fresh lemon juice
2 tbsp soya milk (or rice milk)

Preheat oven to 400°F/200°C/Gas Mark 6. Mix together dry ingredients and rub in butter. Beat in eggs and lemon juice and add sufficient soya milk to make a stiff dropping mixture. Use a tablespoon to drop rough heaps on a greased baking tray. Bake for 8 minutes then cool on a wire tray.

** Corn Cakes

GLUTEN-FREE

125g/4oz/1 scant cup brown rice flour
165g/5½oz/1 cup fine maize meal
2 tsp potassium (or sodium) bicarbonate
65g/2½oz/⅓ cup unsalted butter (or 2½ tbsp unrefined sunflower oil)
240ml/8fl oz/1 cup soya milk (or rice milk)
1 free-range egg
4 tsp fresh lemon juice

Preheat oven to 400°F/200°C/Gas Mark 6. Sift together dry ingredients and rub in butter or oil. Beat together soya milk, egg and lemon juice and stir into flour mixture. Turn into a slightly greased 20cm/8-inch square baking tin and bake for 25 minutes. Test with a knife in the centre. Cut into 5cm/2-inch squares and serve warm with a spread (*see pages 103–9*).

** Millet Buns

GLUTEN-FREE

200g/7oz/1 cup millet grains, ground into flour
1 tsp potassium (or sodium) bicarbonate
25g/1oz unsalted butter (or unhydrogenated margarine)
1 cup grated carrots
2 tsp fresh lemon juice
¾ cup boiling water
3 free-range eggs
2 tbsp cold filtered water

Preheat oven to 375°F/190°C/Gas Mark 5. Mix together the flour and bicarbonate powder, rub in the butter then mix in the carrots and lemon juice. Pour in the boiling water and mix well. Separate the eggs, beat the yolks and add the cold water, then add to the flour mixture. Whisk the egg whites until stiff and fold into the mixture. Butter some tins and spoon the mixture in, not quite to the top. (Muffin tins are deeper than fairy cake tins and are good for this recipe.) Bake for 25 minutes.

** Tea Cakes

225g/8oz/1½ cups plain wholemeal flour
1 tsp potassium (or sodium) bicarbonate
25g/1oz unsalted butter (or unhydrogenated margarine)
1 free-range egg
150ml/¼ pint/⅔ cup soya milk (or rice milk)
2 tsp fresh lemon juice
Sesame seeds for topping

Preheat oven to 375°F/190°C/Gas Mark 5. Sift flour and bicarbonate then rub in the butter. Beat egg, milk and lemon juice together and add to the mixture. Mix to a stiff batter and pour into greased muffin tins (6) or fairy cake tins (12). Sprinkle with sesame seeds and bake for 30 minutes. Cool on a wire tray. Serve with a spread (*pages 103–9*).

Variations

** Beany Tea Cakes

Add dried beans to basic mixture, as many or few as liked.

** Seedy Tea Cakes

Add sunflower seeds to mixture, as many or few as liked.

** Blackcurrant Tea Loaf

550g/1¼lb/4 cups plain wholewheat flour
225g/8oz/1½ cups brown rice flour
2 tsp potassium (or sodium) bicarbonate
2 large carrots, grated
350ml/12fl oz/1½ cups blackcurrant herb tea (use 3 teabags), warm
3 tsp natural vanilla essence
4 tsp fresh lemon juice
1 large tub natural yoghurt

Preheat oven to 400°F/200°C/Gas Mark 6. Mix dry ingredients, then stir in grated carrot. Mix in blackcurrant tea, vanilla essence and lemon juice. Stir in yoghurt – the mixture should be quite moist. Pour into lined tins and bake for 20 minutes at high temperature, then turn tins and bake for a further 20 minutes at reduced temperature (350°F/180°C/Gas Mark 4).

** Squash Muffins

1 large squash, cooked and mashed
300g/12oz/2 cups plain wholemeal flour
2 tsp potassium (or sodium) bicarbonate
⅓ cup unsalted butter
¾ cup natural yoghurt
1 free-range egg
Optional: 1–2 tsp natural vanilla essence or ½ tsp grated nutmeg and ½ tsp ground
  cinnamon

Preheat oven to 375°F/190°C/Gas Mark 5. Cut squash in half lengthways and de-seed. Place halves cut-side down on a lightly greased baking tray and bake for 1 hour until soft (check after 45 minutes). Increase heat to 400°F/200°C/Gas Mark 6. Sift the flour at least three times into a bowl and add dry ingredients. Melt the butter and mix in a separate bowl with the yoghurt and beaten egg. Mix contents of two bowls together, blending with a fork, gently and not too much. Mash the squash and fold into the mixture, together with any optional flavourings. Put into muffin cases and bake for 20–25 minutes. Muffins make a good alternative to soda bread, and taste great with lemon curd (*see page 109*).

Chapter 13

Pastries and Crumble Toppings

The following recipes can be used with many other recipes elsewhere in the book which refer to pastry or a crumble topping. It's good to have a variety of choice.

** (*) Basic Shortcrust Pastry

The success of this pastry depends on correct proportions, and the amounts given below are for one basic measure. For larger pies or flan bases you would need to double or treble these basic amounts. I have to confess that I was never any good at making pastry till I was given a food processor, since when I have found that this recipe never fails to make a completely satisfactory pie crust or flan base, and enables the recipe to have an alternative * category.

3 heaped tbsp plain wholemeal flour
2 heaped tbsp fine or medium oatmeal
2 tbsp unrefined sunflower oil
Filtered water to mix
Optional (for a softer pastry):
I tsp potassium (or sodium) bicarbonate
2 tsp fresh lemon juice

Mix together the dry ingredients, and mix in the oil (and lemon juice, if optional bicarbonate powder is being used). Add water till you have a very sticky dough which just holds together. (In a processor, it suddenly forms a ball.) Coat with plenty of flour for handling, but the wetter the dough the better. Roll out on a floured surface (roll more thinly if using bicarbonate powder).

** Oaty Pastry

75g/3oz/1 cup porridge oats
125g/4oz/1 scant cup plain wholemeal flour
½ tsp potassium (or sodium) bicarbonate
75g/3oz/⅓ cup unsalted butter (or 3 tbsp unrefined sunflower oil)
1 tsp fresh lemon juice
1 free-range egg

Mix together oats, flour and bicarbonate powder, rub in the butter and add the lemon juice. Separate the egg by breaking into a saucer, holding an upturned egg cup over the yolk and allowing the white to run into a cup. Lightly whisk the egg white with a fork and stir into the oaty mixture, adding a few spoonfuls of cold filtered water to form a pliable dough. Knead lightly on a floured surface and press out to 6mm/ ¼-inch thickness.

** Oaty Pasties

The above pastry is good for pasties, containing either meat and vegetables or beans and vegetables. Preheat oven at 400°F/200°C/Gas Mark 6. Having prepared a filling, you cut the pastry into 10cm/4-inch circles, place the filling in the centre, brush water round the edge, bring the edges together at the top and crimp with your finger and thumb to seal. The egg yolk, beaten with 1 tbsp cold filtered water, can be used to brush a glaze over the pasties before they go in the oven. Bake for 20–25 minutes.

** Blind-baked Quiche or Flan Case

This is done incredibly quickly in a microwave. Make one measure of the Basic Shortcrust Pastry, and roll it out to fit a 25cm/10-inch china or glassware flan dish. Prick the bottom all over with a fork, then cover the centre with two pieces of kitchen roll and cover the edges with narrow strips of tin foil (yes, tin foil!). Microwave on High for 4 minutes, remove the paper and foil and microwave again for 2 minutes. When you have put in the filling, you can either microwave on high for 10 minutes, or bake in a pre-heated oven at 350°F/180°C/Gas Mark 4 for 30–40 minutes. Alternatively, you can blind-bake the case in the oven at the same temperature for 20 minutes before adding the filling and completing as before.

** Potato Base

GLUTEN-FREE

Mashed cooked potato mixed with 25g/1oz whole rice flour or soya flour makes a good 'mock pastry' base for a quiche which is gluten-free. Simply mash sufficient potato to line the base and sides of the flan tin, and stir in whichever flour you are using. If gluten is not a problem, this can be plain wholemeal flour.

---

* Basic Crumble Topping 1

WHEAT-FREE

1 mug oats
1 tbsp unrefined sunflower oil or extra virgin olive oil
1 tbsp sesame or sunflower seeds
Optional: 1 tsp mixed dried herbs

Preheat oven to 375°F/190°C/Gas Mark 5. Mix together all ingredients. Sprinkle on top of the filling and bake for 25–30 minutes, depending on the filling.

** Crumble Topping 2

50g/2oz/¼ cup unsalted butter
75g/3oz/½ cup plain wholewheat flour
75g/3oz/1 cup porridge oats
2 tbsp unrefined sunflower oil or extra virgin olive oil
Optional: ½ tsp mixed dried herbs

Preheat the oven to 375°F/190°C/Gas Mark 5. Rub the butter into the flour, stir in the oats and then the oil. Add herbs if using. This mixture can be sprinkled on top of the filling and baked for 25–30 minutes, depending on the filling.

---

* Millet Crumble Topping

GLUTEN-FREE

125g/4oz millet (or millet flakes)
2 cups filtered water
50g/2oz/⅔ cup desiccated coconut (or freshly cracked and ground nuts)

Put millet and water in saucepan over moderate heat, and simmer without stirring. When water has been absorbed, turn off heat and place lid on saucepan, allowing mixture to steam. Leave to cool, then add coconut or ground nuts. Use in place of crumble topping for any recipe.

** Gluten-Free Pastry *(see also pages 265–6)*

150g/5oz/1 cup brown rice flour
75g/3oz/½ cup soya flour
2 tbsp unrefined sunflower oil
Filtered water to mix

Preheat oven to 375°F/190°C/Gas Mark 5. Mix dry ingredients, add oil and mix with fork. Add water to form dough. This pastry is tricky to roll so you might like to do it between two pieces of greaseproof paper. Sprinkle the lower piece with rice flour, place dough on it, then put a second piece of greaseproof paper on top and flatten with a rolling pin. When it is rolled, remove top piece of paper and carry dough to dish on bottom piece of paper. Invert dish on to it, then turn dish right way up, allowing pastry to fall into it. Push into shape. Alternatively, you can roll it out carefully using plenty of soya flour. Prick well all over then blind-bake for about 25 minutes until set but not hard. Use with quiche or flan filling.

Erica White's Beat Candida Cookbook

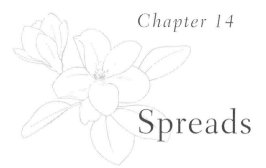

Chapter 14

Spreads

'What on earth can I put on my soda bread or rice cakes?' is a very common cry. Let's talk first of all about the pros and cons of butter and margarine.

From the point of view of starving candida, margarine is slightly better than butter because butter contains lactose – natural milk sugar. However, I do allow a small amount of butter because from all other points of view it is considerably better than the majority of margarines available in the shops, and preferable to most oils – even good quality ones – for cooking. Let me explain.

Fats and oils come in three types – saturated (mainly animal fats, including butter), polyunsaturated (seed and fish oils) and mono-unsaturated (olive oil). Too much saturated fat leads to heart disease and inflammatory conditions in the body and also upsets hormone function, so margarine manufacturers like to claim that their products are made from polyunsaturated oils, like sunflower seeds. Unfortunately, they frequently neglect to point out that their product has turned polyunsaturated oils into a spreading consistency by a process of hydrogenation, and this has the effect of making the oils even more harmful than animal fats!

Probably the very best product from all points of view is an unhydrogenated margarine, but even some of these contain potentially harmful additives and preservatives so you have to read the labels very carefully indeed. There are some good brands available, but you need to buy them from a health-food store rather than a supermarket. Butter is certainly better than a risky margarine.

In addition, when polyunsaturated oils are heated to high temperatures, as in frying or roasting, they produce nasty molecules called free radicals, which attack our bodies and cause a chain reaction of damaged cells. Research increasingly associates free-radical damage with many illnesses from allergies to heart disease, cancer and premature ageing. It is therefore important to consider carefully which oils and fats we use for cooking.

Strangely enough, it is the saturated fats like butter which are safest to use for cooking at high temperatures because they are less prone to free-radical activity than polyunsaturated fats. Olive oil is nearly as stable as butter and this is why you will find that the recipes in this book contain only butter or olive oil for frying or roasting – not that I recommend you to fry or roast very much at all! Oil used for baking does not reach such very high temperatures as it does for roasting or frying, so it is possible to use sunflower oil or unhydrogenated margarine for baking purposes.

It is this problem of free radicals which also makes it important for us to choose cold-pressed, unrefined and extra-virgin oils for salad dressings. We have to have some polyunsaturated oils in our diet, but they should be of a good quality. Any process of oil-extraction other than cold-pressing will have involved heat, and this means that the oil in the bottle will already contain some free radicals. In nature, vitamin E is always found in plants which produce oil because it is an antioxidant – nature's way of preventing free-radical activity. However, cheaper oils have had their vitamin E removed so, if you use these but want to protect yourself from free-radical attack, you should take a daily vitamin E supplement or else squeeze some vitamin E out of the capsules into the bottle of oil so that it will be more like nature intended!

So, back to our discussion of whether or not to use butter; if you don't have an intolerance to cow's milk products, you may use either a little butter as a spread or else a good unhydrogenated margarine. (It will be clearly stated on the label.) Apart from this, the following ideas for spread should help to fill you up. I include cottage cheese, but this must depend on two things. The first is that you are not intolerant to dairy products (this applies equally to butter). Secondly, it depends on how well you are winning the candida war whilst having the small amount of lactose which occurs in cottage cheese. So try it, but be prepared to give it up if your progress seems rather slow – or if you suffer from catarrh or congested sinuses, because all cow's milk products increase the production of mucus.

* Quick Spreads

Cottage cheese (possibly); tinned fish – mashed; avocado – mashed; hummus – home-made *(see page 106)* or shop-bought, but make sure it contains no vinegar or citric acid; chicken jelly – saved from the pan with any fat removed; olive pâté from your health-food store; canned beans – mashed. With any of these you could have sliced tomatoes, cucumber, chives, cress or watercress.

Quick Spreads

The following spreads are quick and easy to make yourself, but the seedy butters do need a electric grinder.

* Seedy Butter

GLUTEN-FREE

Grind any seeds, or mixture of seeds, till they are powdery. Keep in a jar in the refrigerator, remove a quantity as needed and mix with a very small amount of filtered water to form a paste. Try sunflower seeds, pumpkin seeds, flax (linseeds) and sesame seeds; a mixture of sunflower and sesame tastes good. You can also lightly toast half of the seeds in a dry frying pan, which gives a different flavour. It is possible to buy sunflower seed spread and tahini (sesame seed spread) ready-made from roasted seeds, but when I suffered from candida in the mouth I found that these products caused a flare-up of the symptoms, which probably meant that they contained a degree of mould, rather like peanut butter.

* Carob Seedy Butter

GLUTEN-FREE

To 1 cup of ground seeds (not toasted), add 1 or 2 teaspoons of carob powder, according to taste, mix with water as above and you have a healthy alternative to chocolate spread.

** Hummus 1

GLUTEN-FREE

200g/7oz/1 cup chickpeas (garbanzos), soaked overnight and boiled for 1 hour OR
1 can sugar-free chickpeas (garbanzos), rinsed to remove salt
2 lemons, squeezed
1 tbsp extra virgin olive oil
1 garlic clove, crushed
90g/3oz/¾ cup ground sesame seeds

Drain and rinse chickpeas (garbanzos), purée in a blender with the lemon juice and oil or press through a sieve. Add garlic and ground sesame seeds, and mix to a thick paste, adding water if necessary. Keep refrigerated.

Hummus 2

GLUTEN-FREE

1 can sugar-free chickpeas (garbanzos), rinsed to remove salt
½–1 tsp garlic granules, according to preference
150ml/¼ pint/⅔ cup natural low-fat yoghurt
½ lemon, squeezed

Mix all ingredients in processor or blender; leave slightly lumpy.

** Lentil Pâté

GLUTEN-FREE

1 medium onion
1 clove garlic
2 tbsp extra virgin olive oil
125g/4oz/⅔ cup lentils

600ml/1 pint/2½ cups yeast-free vegetable stock (see *page 126*)
½ tsp ground turmeric
½ tsp ground coriander
½ tsp ground cumin

Chop onion and garlic and soften in oil in a deep pan. Rinse lentils and add to pan. Pour in stock and add spices. Bring to the boil and then turn down heat to a gentle simmer until lentils are soft and the mixture is thick. Remove from heat, leave to cool and then beat with a wooden spoon to make a paste, or alternatively use an electric blender.

Variation: tomato pâté can be made in the same way by omitting the spices and adding 1 tbsp of tomato purée.

---

* Beany Spread

GLUTEN-FREE

125g/4oz/⅔ cup haricot beans, soaked and cooked (see *page 168*) OR
1 can ready-cooked haricot beans or others (no sugar)
25g/1oz unsalted butter (or 1 tbsp unrefined sunflower oil)
3 tbsp chopped parsley
2 cloves garlic, crushed (or 1 tsp garlic granules)
2 tbsp tomato purée (no citric acid)
Optional: freshly ground black pepper

Mash the beans to a smooth paste, or use processor. Slightly soften the butter, then blend into beans with all other ingredients. Chill until required.

---

* Tuna Spread 1

GLUTEN-FREE

1 small can tuna in brine, drained
250g/8oz/1 cup cottage cheese
1 tbsp chopped fresh chives
Squeeze of fresh lemon juice

Mix all ingredients to smooth paste, or use processor or blender. Chill until required.

---

* Tuna Spread 2

GLUTEN-FREE

2 large carrots (or 1 carrot and 1 parsnip), peeled and chopped
1 large onion, chopped
1 small can tuna in brine, drained

Simmer carrots (or carrot and parsnip) and onion in a very little water until soft, and liquid is reduced to 2 tbsp. Mash well and mix in tuna.

---

* Avocado Spread

GLUTEN-FREE

2 ripe avocados
1 ripe tomato, peeled
2 tbsp fresh lemon juice
1 tbsp chopped chives
1 clove garlic crushed (or ½ tsp garlic granules)
Optional: pinch of any herb

Mash and mix all ingredients, or use blender. Chill until required.

Tofu Spreads

The foregoing recipes can be stretched to go further and also given a high protein content and creamy consistency by the addition of 50g/2oz of tofu, which is soya bean curd and can be bought in blocks. (Don't buy the smoked variety.) Another tofu spread is given below:

* Basic Tofu Spread

GLUTEN-FREE

300g/10oz tofu
1 tbsp tomato purée (no citric acid)
½ tsp garlic granules
Pinch of dried basil
Freshly ground black pepper

Mix or blend all the ingredients until smooth.

* Lemon Curd

GLUTEN-FREE

25g/1oz/knob unsalted butter
1 organic lemon
1 free-range egg

Melt butter in a basin over a pan of boiling water. When soft, remove from heat and grate the rind of a well-scrubbed lemon into the melted butter, then squeeze the lemon and add the juice. Beat with a wooden spoon, then add an egg and continue to beat. Return basin to heat over the pan and stir constantly until mixture thickens. Good with Squash Muffins *(page 98)*, various scones *(pages 91–5)* or American Pancakes *(pages 238–9)* as a tea-time treat or dessert.

Chapter 15

Dips and Savoury Snacks

M any of the recipes given in this chapter are useful as spreads or as pancake fillers. They also make a simple and healthy treat if used as dips with vegetable crudités. Most of these recipes require a blender. What can you use for crudités? The answer to that is, 'Almost anything'. Here are a few ideas to get you started:

* Crudités

Many raw vegetables are suitable, e.g. carrots, celery, cucumber, cauliflower, peppers, radishes, swedes, mooli (long white radishes). You can cut some into matchsticks, some into rings or slices, and cauliflower of course makes pretty florets. Choose three or four with contrasting colours and use a variety of shapes.

Dips

* Hummus *(see 'Spreads', page 106)*

* Sunflower Dip

GLUTEN-FREE

125g/4oz/1 cup sunflower seeds
½ tsp garlic granules
1 stick celery, finely chopped
Juice of ½ lemon

Blend all ingredients in liquidizer till smooth.

* Avocado and Tofu Dip

-GLUTEN-FREE

1 ripe avocado
150g/5oz tofu (soya bean curd)
Juice of ½ lemon
½ tsp garlic granules
2 tbsp soya milk, if needed

Blend all ingredients in liquidizer till smooth.

* Avocado and Tuna Dip

GLUTEN-FREE

1 small can tuna (in brine), rinsed
1 ripe avocado, peeled and stoned
1 small tub natural low-fat yoghurt
Juice of ½ lemon

Blend all ingredients in liquidizer till smooth.

* Avocado and Lemon Dip

GLUTEN-FREE

I ripe avocado
Juice of ½ lemon
5 tbsp natural low-fat yoghurt
I tsp ground coriander

Blend all ingredients in liquidizer till smooth.

* Avocado and Tomato Dip

GLUTEN-FREE

2 ripe avocados
I large tomato, peeled
4 tsp fresh lemon juice
I tbsp chopped chives (or spring onions/scallions)
½ tsp garlic granules (or I clove garlic, crushed)

Peel and mash avocados and tomato and thoroughly mix with other ingredients.

* Yoghurt and Cucumber Dip

GLUTEN-FREE

I small cucumber
I small tub natural low-fat yoghurt
I tsp garlic granules (or 2 cloves garlic, crushed)
I tsp fresh lemon juice
I tsp mint, finely chopped

Peel cucumber, grate in a processor and press out liquid through a sieve. Mix the flesh with other ingredients. Chill till required.

* Yoghurt and Tuna Dip

GLUTEN-FREE

1 small can tuna in brine, rinsed
1 small tub natural low-fat yoghurt

Mix together well with a fork.

* Salmon (or Tuna) and Cottage Cheese Dip

GLUTEN-FREE

340g/12oz/1½ cups cottage cheese
1 small can salmon or tuna in brine (rinsed)
1 tbsp chopped chives (or spring onion/scallion)
1 tbsp chopped parsley
1 tsp fresh lemon juice

Mix together well with a fork or in liquidizer.

* Tahini Dip

GLUTEN-FREE

1 small tub natural low-fat yoghurt
60g/2oz/½ cup ground sesame seeds, with a little water to make a runny paste
1 tsp fresh lemon juice
½ tsp garlic granules (or 1 clove garlic, crushed)

Mix well together or liquidize in blender.

* Red Bean Dip

GLUTEN-FREE

This dip formed part of a delicious lunch-time spread provided by a client whilst I was on a lecture tour in Dubai. I associate it with blue skies and spacious, cool houses.

1 can red kidney beans (sugar-free), rinsed
1 tbsp fresh lemon juice
1 clove of garlic
1 tbsp extra virgin olive oil
1 tbsp tomato purée

Thoroughly drain and rinse the beans. Put all ingredients in a food processor and whizz. Each of the ingredients may be adjusted to taste.

Savoury Snacks

Apart from dips, what other sorts of savoury snacks can you have? Well, there are any of the 'Spreads' (*Chapter 14*) with any of the soda breads or whole-grain biscuits, like oat-cakes, rice cakes or crispbreads. For a hot lunch-time snack, you could toast some soda bread and have poached or scrambled egg on it, or grilled tomatoes, or sardines. You can buy instant wholewheat noodles which you leave to stand for just four minutes in boiling water – very useful for a quick and easy spaghetti-type dish.

* Home-made Popcorn

GLUTEN-FREE

Home-made popcorn is one of the cheapest, easiest snacks to make, and a habit which is difficult to stop once you've started eating it!

Knob of unsalted butter
1 tbsp popping corn

Choose a large saucepan with a well-fitting lid, and melt a very small knob of butter over medium heat. Put in the corn and fit the lid on the saucepan tightly. In just a few moments you will hear the corn start popping. Shake the saucepan frequently, and remove from the heat when the popping has stopped. Empty quickly into a bowl to cool.

It is possible to make popcorn in a microwave without using butter, in a dish with a well-fitting lid. I find it takes longer than in a saucepan, but it does avoid the fat.

Do not try to re-cook any grains which have not 'popped'.

---

* Tomato and Tuna Topping

GLUTEN-FREE

The following recipe is a topping which you could have on toast, baked potato or whole-wheat pasta.

2 tsp tomato purée
150ml/¼ pt/⅔ cup water
1 small onion, chopped
1 small can tuna in brine (rinsed)
Pinch of oregano

Mix tomato purée with the water, add onion and cook over low heat for a few minutes until onion is soft. Flake the tuna and add it with oregano to the pan. Cook until heated through and liquid has reduced a little.

---

* Wholemeal Garlic Bread

If garlic bread is a favourite of yours, try making it with the Yoghurt Soda Bread recipe (*see page 73*). It takes a lot of butter, so don't have it too often!

Unsalted butter to spread
Crushed garlic cloves (allow 1 per person)
Mixed herbs
1 Yoghurt Soda Bread loaf (*see page 73*), preferably cooked in a tin and cut into
    12mm/½-inch slices

Melt butter in a pan. Add garlic and herbs. Spread the butter on the sliced bread and put slices back together before putting into a covered casserole dish. (Use foil if you don't have the right sized dish.) Heat in oven at 300°F/150°C/Gas Mark 2 for 15–20 minutes.

Snacks and Lunch-box Fillers

The following recipes make useful snacks or lunch-box fillers, so it would be worth making a batch for your freezer.

** Pizza

1 batch Basic Shortcrust Pastry (see page 99)
1 clove garlic
1 onion
900g/2lb/5 cups tomatoes
1 tbsp soya flour (or brown rice flour)
1 tsp dried oregano
Freshly ground black pepper
Rings of coloured peppers and onion to decorate

Preheat oven to 350°F/180°C/Gas Mark 4. Roll out pastry to slightly larger than a pie plate, lay on plate and trim roughly, using surplus to make a lip round the edge. Process the garlic, onion and tomatoes in a blender, add the flour and blend again. Spread the sauce over the pastry, sprinkle with oregano and black pepper. Decorate with rings of coloured peppers and onion. Bake for 25 minutes. (Alternatively, you can add the peppers and onion rings just before serving, so they are served raw on top of the pizza.)

** Pizza Scones

225g/8oz/1½ cups plain wholemeal flour
2 tsp potassium (or sodium) bicarbonate
50g/2oz/¼ cup unsalted butter

125ml/4fl oz/½ cup soya milk (or rice milk)
4 tsp fresh lemon juice

Topping:
1 tbsp extra virgin olive oil
1 medium onion, chopped
400g/14oz/2-cup can of tomatoes (no citric acid)
½ tsp mixed dried herbs

Extra topping ideas: prawns, tuna, cottage cheese, sweetcorn, green pepper, cooked chicken.

Preheat oven to 425°F/220°C/Gas Mark 7. Sift dry ingredients and rub in butter. Add soya milk and lemon juice and mix to a soft dough. Knead lightly on floured surface, roll out to 12mm/ ½-inch thickness. Cut out 5cm/2½-inch rounds and place on floured baking sheet. Bake for 10–12 minutes.

While scones are baking, heat the oil in a pan, add the onion and cook gently until soft. Chop the tomatoes and add to pan together with herbs, and cook till sauce is reduced to jam-like consistency. Remove scones from oven, cut in halves and put them back on the baking sheet, cut side up. Put a spoonful of mixture on each and spread it to the edges. Put on any extra toppings, then bake for a further 10–12 minutes.

** Potato Scones

15g/½ oz/knob unsalted butter (or unhydrogenated margarine)
225g/8oz/1⅓ cups cooked potatoes, mashed
50g/2oz/⅓ cup wholemeal flour

Mix butter or margarine with mashed potatoes and work in as much flour as the paste will take up. Roll out thinly, shape into rounds or squares and prick well. Lightly grease a frying pan with a very little olive oil or butter, and fry scones for 3 minutes on each side until browned.

** Sardine Rolls

1 batch of Basic Shortcrust Pastry (see page 99)
1 can sardines, rinsed and drained
Tomato purée (no citric acid)
Freshly ground black pepper
Optional: white of 1 egg for glazing

Preheat oven to 400°F/200°C/Gas Mark 6. Roll out pastry and cut into 10cm/4-inch circles. Mash sardines with tomato purée to taste, season with pepper and place heaped teaspoonful on one half of the pastry circles. Moisten edges with water, and fold pastry over to form a semi-circle. Press the edges together firmly. Brush with white of egg. Bake for 15 minutes.

** Turkey Burgers

450g/1lb/2 cups minced turkey
1 small onion
15g/½ oz/scant ¼ cup crushed rye crispbreads
½ tsp mixed dried herbs
Freshly ground black pepper

Mix all ingredients together and divide into 12 portions. Shape into balls and press into burger shapes on a floured board. Separate with freezer layering film or greaseproof paper and freeze till required. When using, thaw thoroughly and cook both sides under a hot grill.

*** Turkey Rolls

Use the above burger mix and make into sausage rolls using Basic Shortcrust Pastry recipe (see page 99). Cook at 350°F/180°C/Gas Mark 4 for about 30 minutes, till turkey filling is well cooked.

** Bean and Vegetable Pasties

Eat like mince pies at Christmas! Preheat oven to 375°F/190°C/Gas Mark 5. Cook up any bean and vegetable stew mix (*see pages 169–70*) and make a batch of Basic Shortcrust Pastry (*see page 99*). Use bun tray or muffin tins. Line with pastry, add filling, and cover with pastry lid, making a small slit with a knife for steam to escape. Bake for 15 minutes. Cool on a wire tray. Ideally, warm through before eating, otherwise eat cold. Keep a batch in the freezer and pop a couple in the microwave or oven to thaw and warm as needed.

* Chapatti Bread

675g/1½lb/5 cups wholemeal flour
3 tbsp extra virgin olive oil
350ml/12fl oz/1½ cups filtered water
Optional: ½ tsp Lo-salt

Mix ingredients together, cut dough into 10 pieces and roll into circles to fit a frying pan. Cook in hot pan without grease for 30–45 seconds on each side. Makes 8 or 10.

** Sweetcorn Fritters

125g/4oz/1 scant cup wholemeal flour
1 medium free-range egg
150ml/¼pt/⅔ cup water (approximately)
1 small can sweetcorn (sugar-free) or 125g/4oz/½ cup frozen sweetcorn
1 spring onion (scallion), chopped
Extra virgin olive oil for frying
Optional: 125g/4oz/1 scant cup peas, cooked from frozen
Optional: 1 red pepper, finely diced

Mix wholemeal flour, egg and water until you have a smooth batter mixture. Add the vegetables and mix in well. Pour a little olive oil into a frying pan and heat, then drop in spoonfuls of batter and cook until golden brown. Drain on kitchen roll. Eat hot or cold.

---

* Corn Crisps

GLUTEN-FREE

2 tbsp unsalted butter (or extra virgin olive oil)
85g/3oz/½ cup fine maize meal
Optional: ½ tsp Lo-salt
200ml/7fl oz/¾ cup boiling water
Celery seeds or poppy seeds for sprinkling

Preheat oven to 425°F/220°C/Gas Mark 7. Rub the butter or olive oil into the maize meal and optional Lo-salt. Pour in the boiling water, stirring well. Place teaspoonsful of the mixture onto non-stick baking trays, spaced well apart to allow for spreading. Sprinkle with celery or poppy seeds. Bake for 8 minutes, till golden brown. Remove from trays carefully with spatula whilst still hot. Makes 48 x 5cm/2-inch crisps.

Chapter 16

Starters and Appetizers

S oup obviously makes a very good first course, but it deserves – and has been given – a whole chapter to itself (*see Chapter 17*). Similarly, crudités with dips make an interesting start to a meal, and these have been covered in Chapter 15. The following ideas are for hot or cold starters, but can also be used as light snacks in their own right. However, for those who are REVIVING or even THRIVING, these dishes are easy to prepare if you are having friends to dinner and want to serve an interesting first course.

---

* Avocado Pâté 1

GLUTEN-FREE

4 free-range eggs
2 avocados
1 lemon
1 garlic clove, chopped (or ½ tsp garlic granules)
2 tsp chopped mint or lemon balm
Freshly ground black pepper
Optional: parsley, lemon slice, lettuce leaves, to garnish

Hard-boil the eggs in advance, and chop finely when cool. Cut the avocados in half and remove the stones, then remove the flesh to a bowl, leaving the shells intact.

Squeeze half the lemon and add the juice, together with the chopped garlic and all other ingredients. Mash with a fork or liquidize in a blender. Put mixture back into shells, garnish with parsley sprigs or a slice of lemon pushed into the mixture, and arrange on lettuce leaves on individual plates.

---

* Avocado Pâté 2

GLUTEN-FREE

½ can pease pudding
1 avocado
Juice of ½ lemon
Freshly ground black pepper
1 clove garlic, crushed (or 1 tsp garlic granules)

Mash all ingredients together, mixing well. Serve with crudités, soya cookies, oat cakes etc.

---

* Eggs with Avocado Sauce

GLUTEN-FREE

4 free-range eggs
1 soft avocado
3 tbsp natural yoghurt
½ tbsp tomato purée (no citric acid)
4 tbsp chopped parsley
Garnish: lettuce, mustard and cress, tomato

Hard-boil the eggs in advance, remove shells under cold water, leave to cool then cut in half lengthways. Remove the flesh from the avocado and mash or blend with the yoghurt, tomato purée and parsley. Put two egg-halves on a bed of lettuce on individual plates, cover with the avocado sauce, sprinkle with mustard and cress and garnish with slices of tomato.

---

* Prawn and Avocado Salad

175g/6oz/2 cups wholemeal pasta shapes
1 ripe avocado
225g/8oz/2 cups frozen peeled prawns, thawed
1 lemon
2 tbsp unrefined sunflower oil
1 clove garlic, crushed (or ½ tsp garlic granules)
1 tbsp chopped chives

Cook the pasta in a saucepan of boiling water for 10–12 minutes, drain and allow to cool. Cut avocado in half, remove stone and carefully remove shell. Cut the halves into slices, and mix gently with pasta and prawns. Squeeze the lemon and combine juice with oil, garlic and chives in a screw-top jar. Shake well and pour over salad. Alternatively, blend the dressing in a liquidizer.

* Prawn Cocktail

GLUTEN-FREE

¼ iceberg lettuce
225g/8oz/2 cups frozen peeled prawns, thawed
1 small tub Greek yoghurt
Garnish: cucumber slices (cut to centre and twisted), wedge of lemon.
Optional: 1 avocado

Chop lettuce into long, fine strands, and put into the bottom of individual glass dishes. Put a quarter of the prawns into each dish, top with a tablespoon of Greek yoghurt and decorate with a twist of cucumber and wedge of lemon. If using avocado, remove shell and dice the flesh, mixing in gently with the prawns before adding yoghurt.

Hot starters (see below) are very easy to organize if you have a microwave oven, though obviously they could equally be heated through in a conventional oven at medium heat, say 350°F/180°C/Gas Mark 4.

* Hot Pilchards and Yoghurt

GLUTEN-FREE

400g/14oz can of pilchards in brine (or canned mackerel)
175g/6oz/1 cup tomatoes
150ml/¼ pt/⅔ cup natural yoghurt
Garnish: parsley sprigs

Thoroughly rinse the pilchards, remove any bones and mash the fish well. Pour boiling water over the tomatoes to make it easy to remove the skins, then chop and put into the bottom of four small ramekin dishes. Divide the mashed fish and add on top of the tomatoes. Spoon the yoghurt over the fish. Cook in a microwave for 4 minutes on High (or heat in the oven for 10–15 minutes at 350°F/180°C/Gas Mark 4), then decorate with parsley and serve.

* Hot (or Cold) Avocados with Dressing

GLUTEN-FREE

2 ripe avocados
125ml/4fl oz/½ cup natural yoghurt
1 tbsp tomato purée
Garnish: watercress

If using a conventional oven, preheat to 425°F/220°C/Gas Mark 7. Cut the avocados in half and remove the stones. Place in individual china dishes or arrange in one large dish. Mix the yoghurt with the tomato purée and pour over the avocados. Heat in the oven for 10–15 minutes, or cover and cook in the microwave on High for 2 minutes. Decorate with watercress and serve.

This recipe can be varied by putting peeled prawns into the avocado before adding the yoghurt mixture, or by using cottage cheese in place of yoghurt and sprinkling with a little paprika. Any of these variations are just as delicious, in fact, served cold, the combination of yoghurt with tomato purée providing an excellent contrast in flavour with the avocado.

*** Carrot Soufflé

GLUTEN-FREE

340g/12oz/2 cups grated carrots
1 cup finely chopped onions
1 tbsp unrefined sunflower oil
1 free-range egg
Pinch of powdered cloves
Garnish: cucumber, watercress etc.

Preheat oven to 350°F/180°C/Gas Mark 4. Steam grated carrots until really soft and soften onions in the oil over a low heat or in the microwave. Purée together in a blender. Separate the egg by breaking it into a saucer and holding an egg-cup over the yolk, then pouring off the white into a bowl. Add the yolk to the blender and mix in well. Whisk the egg-white until stiff, and fold it into the carrot mixture. Add a pinch of cloves. Spoon mixture into a buttered loaf tin and bake for 20–25 minutes. Serve in hot slices, decorated with any available garnish.

* Chicken Liver Pâté

GLUTEN-FREE

2 large onions
2 tbsp extra virgin olive oil
225g/8oz/1 cup chicken livers
2 tsp dried mixed herbs
2 tbsp tomato purée
1–2 tbsp soya milk (or rice milk), to blend

Finely chop onions and soften in the oil over a low heat. Clean and chop the livers, add to onions and cook for 5 minutes, stirring well. Reduce heat and add herbs. Cover pan and cook gently for 20 minutes, stirring occasionally, until liver is completely cooked. Place in blender with tomato purée and mix to a smooth paste. Add a little soya milk if mixture is too

Chapter 17

Stocks, Soups and Gravies

The very easiest way to obtain a stock or a soup is to buy soya cubes from a health-food shop. This is ideal for a SURVIVOR, provided you have some-one to do the shopping! There are various stock or bouillon cubes available, but the vast majority seem to contain yeast, so do read the labels carefully. Most are also high in salt, so they are not in fact the most healthy way of making stock or soup.

For a warming tomato soup, there is nothing easier than opening a packet of tomato juice (free of citric acid) and heating it through in a saucepan, or in a mug in the microwave. It tastes so delicious that I wonder why the tomato soup you buy needs to have so many other ingredients!

Vegetable Stock

Saving the water from cooked vegetables is an excellent way of obtaining nourishing stock. One thrifty client always saves this water in yoghurt cartons and puts it in the freezer till needed, thereby always having some stock to add to recipes. Of course, if you steam your vegetables, as you really should in order not to lose all their nutrients, there will not be a great deal of water to save, but what little you do have is extremely nourishing, having taken up many of the nutrients lost by the vegetables in the cooking process.

Vegetable stock is also easily made from the discarded bits of prepared vegetables, like carrot ends and outer cabbage leaves, preferably organic. Wash them thoroughly and chop them, put into a large pan and just cover with water, bring to the boil and simmer for 15 minutes. Strain off the liquid, cool and freeze.

Chicken Stock

Another client always has a similar supply of chicken stock to hand. She says, 'Whenever I cook a chicken, I keep the carcass and make up a good stock the next day. Then I freeze the stock in 150ml/¼-pint/⅔-cup, 300ml/½-pint/1⅓-cup and 600ml/1-pint/2½-cup portions, and it's simply a matter of defrosting it to add wonderful flavour to soups, risottos, etc.'

To make stock from cooked chicken bones, cover the bones with water, bring to the boil and simmer for 30 minutes. (If using raw bones, this should be three hours, or else half an hour in a pressure cooker.) Strain off the liquid and allow to cool, then remove the fat from the top. Freeze the stock in containers.

Gravies

These can also be kept in ready supply in the freezer by making purées from any mixture of vegetables. The vegetables should be cooked together until soft and then put through a blender. Different vegetables go well with different meals – experiment with whatever is available and see which combinations you prefer. It's a good idea to cook more vegetables than you need for a particular meal, then purée the leftovers and freeze. Heated through, this makes a thick and savoury sauce.

Puréed vegetables are a good way of thickening any stock to make it into a broth or thick soup, so there is no end to the variety of flavours you can create just by using leftovers and discarded bits of vegetables.

However, I have been sent some very tasty recipes using particular ingredients, and they are too delicious not to include. The first one is described by a client as the simplest, most delicious soup ever!

* Butternut Squash Soup

GLUTEN-FREE, SERVES 2

1 medium butternut squash
500ml/¾ pint/2¼ cups vegetable stock
Freshly ground black pepper
Freshly grated nutmeg

Preheat oven to 375°F/190°/Gas Mark 5. Cut squash in half lengthways and de-seed. Place halves cut-side down on a lightly greased baking tray and bake for 1 hour until soft (check after 45 minutes). Allow to cool then scoop out the flesh and blend with the stock in a liquidizer until smooth. Pour into saucepan and reheat gently. Season with pepper and nutmeg to taste.

Potato Soups

Potato makes a good basis for thick winter-warming broths, but you need to be aware that when it is overcooked it is digested into glucose very quickly. For all that, it is a useful, filling and nutritious vegetable, and its hypoglycaemic effect can largely be counteracted if you make sure you eat some fibre (from whole grains or raw vegetable salad) at the same meal. So here are recipes using potato as their base.

** Watercress and Potato Soup

GLUTEN-FREE

900ml/1½ pints/3¾ cups home-made chicken stock
2 small onions or shallots
350g/12oz/2½ cups diced potatoes
175g/6oz/6 cups chopped watercress
125ml/4fl oz/½ cup natural yoghurt
Pinch of herbs
Freshly ground black pepper

Put stock, onions and potatoes into a large pan. Bring to the boil, cover and simmer for 10 minutes. Stir in the watercress and yoghurt, and simmer for a further 5 minutes. Liquidize in a blender or food processor. Season with a pinch of favourite herbs or black pepper, reheat and serve.

This recipe can be varied in many ways. For instance, you can use leeks instead of onions, courgettes (zucchini) instead of potatoes, parsley instead of watercress, a tin of tomatoes (mashed) instead of yoghurt. Have fun!

---

* Leek and Potato Soup 1

GLUTEN-FREE

1 large potato, scrubbed but not peeled
1 large leek, scrubbed
900ml/1½ pints/3¾ cups water
Herbs to season
Freshly ground black pepper
2 tbsp soya milk (or rice milk)

Chop vegetables, cover with water and bring to boil. Simmer for 15–20 minutes. This can be served as it is or put through a blender. Just before serving, stir in the soya milk.

---

* Leek and Potato Soup 2

GLUTEN-FREE

4 large potatoes, scrubbed and chopped
1½ mugs frozen leeks
1 yeast-free stock cube, or pinch of Lo-salt
Freshly ground black pepper
2 tsp dried chives (or 2 tbsp chopped fresh chives)
½ tsp dried mixed herbs

Place all the ingredients in a large saucepan. Cover with water. Bring to the boil, cover and simmer over a low heat until vegetables are soft. Blend in liquidizer till smooth.

---

* Potato and Broccoli Soup

GLUTEN-FREE

3 large potatoes
3 sticks of celery
1 head of broccoli
1–2 tbsp extra virgin olive oil
900ml/1½ pints/3¾ cups filtered water
Freshly ground black pepper

Peel and cube potatoes. Wash celery and broccoli and slice into small pieces. Put all vegetables into a large pan with the olive oil and sauté for 15 minutes. Add the water and lightly season with the pepper, bring to the boil and simmer for 20 minutes. Blend in the liquidizer.

Other Vegetable Soups

Parsnips are rather similar to potatoes in their usefulness as a base for thick soups, and these also should be eaten with a meal containing fibre.

* Parsnip Soup

GLUTEN-FREE

450g/1 lb/3½ cups parsnips, peeled and roughly chopped
1 large onion, roughly chopped
½ tsp cumin powder
½ tsp coriander powder
600ml/1 pint/2½ cups water (up to twice this amount for thinner soup)
4 tbsp natural yoghurt

Place all ingredients except yoghurt into a large saucepan and simmer until vegetables are soft. Put through a blender, pour into dishes and swirl a spoonful of yoghurt round the top of each, as a garnish.

* Leek and Parsnip Soup

GLUTEN-FREE

This recipe is similar to the previous one, but uses leeks instead of onion and chicken stock instead of water.

1 large parsnip, peeled and chopped
2–3 leeks, scrubbed and chopped
600ml/1 pint/2½ cups home-made chicken stock
1 tbsp chickpea flour (gram flour)
Freshly ground black pepper
Herbs to taste

Put the chopped vegetables into a large pan with the stock, bring to the boil and simmer till soft. Put through a blender, thicken with chickpea flour and return to heat, stirring all the time. Add pepper and herbs.

** Yellow Winter Soup

GLUTEN-FREE

Dried peas and lentils make a good thickening base to a soup and also add to its protein content.

175g/6oz/¾ cup split dried peas
175g/6oz/1¼ cups carrots
175g/6oz/1¼ cups swede
1 medium onion
1 tbsp extra virgin olive oil
900ml/1½ pints/3¾ cups home-made chicken stock
Freshly ground black pepper
Herbs to taste

Wash the split peas and soak them overnight in cold water. Drain before use. Chop all the vegetables. Soften the onion in the oil over a low heat, add carrots and swede and continue to cook over gentle heat for 5 minutes. Add the split peas and chicken stock.

Cover, bring to the boil and simmer for 1½ hours until peas are really soft. Season to taste.

---

* Nutmeg Carrot Soup

GLUTEN-FREE

25g/1oz/knob unsalted butter (or 1 tbsp extra virgin olive oil)
450g/1lb/3¼ cups carrots
1 large potato
1 medium onion
600ml/1 pint/2½ cups vegetable stock
25g/1oz whole-grain rice
Freshly ground nutmeg
Freshly ground black pepper
2 tsp lemon juice

Peel and coarsely grate the carrots and potato, then grate the onion. (A food processor grater attachment is ideal.) Melt butter or oil in a large pan over a low heat and add the grated vegetables. Cook for 5 minutes then add the stock, rice, large pinch of nutmeg and black pepper if required. Bring to the boil, then simmer for 45 minutes. Add lemon juice and serve in 4 bowls, with more nutmeg grated on top.

---

* Tomato, Carrot and Lentil Soup

GLUTEN-FREE

2 large onions, chopped
400g/14oz/2-cup can tomatoes (or fresh tomatoes)
4 medium carrots, grated
1.2 litres/2 pints/5 cups liquid (water, stock or half of each)
4 tsp tomato purée (no citric acid)
150g/5oz/¾ cup split red lentils
1 bay leaf
1 level tsp turmeric

1 heaped tsp cumin
Freshly ground black pepper to taste

Soften the onions, tomatoes and carrots in the liquid and tomato purée for 5 minutes over a gentle heat. Add lentils, spices and seasoning. Cover and bring to the boil. Turn down heat and simmer for 40 minutes. Serve chunky or put through a blender. This client comments, 'Especially delicious served with toasted soda bread!' A similar recipe includes 'a couple of handfuls of brown rice' to make 'a wonderfully quick, easy and satis-fying meal – a life-saver for me!'.

* Cream of Tomato Soup

GLUTEN-FREE

2 large potatoes, scrubbed and chopped
1 can tomatoes
2 tbsp tomato purée (no citric acid)
½ tsp dried basil
1 tsp dried mixed herbs
1 tsp paprika
Pinch of Lo-salt
1 mug soya milk (or rice milk)
Juice of 1 lemon

Place all ingredients except lemon juice into a large saucepan. Bring to boil, cover and simmer until potatoes are soft. The soya milk may appear curdled but this will be blend-ed in. Blend in liquidizer until smooth, adding lemon juice to taste.

* Pressure-Cooked Minestrone

GLUTEN-FREE

If you have a pressure cooker, vegetable soups are particularly easy.
Collect together as many different vegetables as you can lay hands on – 1 medium carrot, 1 small turnip, 2 sticks celery, 1 medium leek, 2 tomatoes, quarter cabbage, 1 medium potato. Any others would be equally acceptable! Chop them all up into cubes

(shred the cabbage), and to these you need to add the following ingredients:

1 medium onion, chopped
1 clove garlic, crushed
1 tbsp extra virgin olive oil
4 tsp chopped parsley
4 tsp tomato purée (no citric acid)
900ml/1½ pints/3¾ cups hot vegetable stock
25g/1oz/⅓ cup wholewheat spaghetti, broken into short lengths

Gently fry onion and garlic in oil in the pressure cooker for 1 minute. Add all vegetables except tomatoes and cabbage, and cook gently for 5 minutes. Add tomatoes, tomato purée, cabbage and stock, bring to the boil and add spaghetti. Stir well and close the cooker. Bring to High pressure and cook for 8 minutes. Reduce pressure quickly.

---

* Cauliflower Soup

GLUTEN-FREE

1 medium onion
900ml/1½ pints/3¾ cups water
1 cauliflower
2 sticks of celery
1–2 tbsp extra virgin olive oil
1 handful fresh parsley, chopped
Freshly grated nutmeg
Freshly ground black pepper

Chop onion and sauté in oil until transparent. Add the water and bring to the boil, then add all the other ingredients. Simmer for 20 minutes and liquidize in a blender.

Chilled Soup

To make an interesting change from hot soups, how about trying a chilled soup in the summer? It would make a good talking-point at your dinner party, yet rates only a * energy level.

---

* Chilled Soup

GLUTEN-FREE

1 medium onion, chopped
2 tbsp extra virgin olive oil
2 bunches watercress, washed and chopped
600ml/1 pint/2½ cups vegetable stock
300ml/½ pint/1⅓ cups natural yoghurt

Soften the onion in the oil for a few minutes. Add watercress, stirring all the time. After 2 minutes add the stock and bring to the boil. Cover and simmer for 20 minutes. Allow to cool and put through a blender. Leave in the refrigerator for at least 2 hours. Just before serving, return to blender with the yoghurt. This would look good served with a sprig of watercress on top.

Chapter 18

Salads and Dressings

R aw vegetables offer the best value in terms of nutrients, and also provide tremendous variety, yet we so seldom think of salad as anything other than lettuce with cucumber and tomatoes. Even lettuce can offer variety: cos, iceberg, salad bowl and round or cabbage lettuce all have a slightly different flavour and texture. Then there are endive and Chinese leaves. You can use white or red cabbage as a salad base, but not many people seem to think of using spinach leaves. Watercress and mustard-and-cress both bring variety to flavour and appearance, and you might also like to try nasturtium leaves from the garden. Grated Brussels sprouts bring an interesting flavour to a mixed green salad, as do chopped celery and mangetout peas, complete with their pods.

When and where possible, and if you can afford it, buy organic produce to reduce your intake of pesticides and other pollutants, and so reduce the toxic load on your immune system and liver. The pollution factor is so severe that, in one year, the average person breathes in two grams of solid pollutants and eats twelve pounds of chemical food additives as well as a gallon of pesticides. If you do not have a local supplier of organic produce, or cannot afford to buy it, make sure that you thoroughly wash all vegetables which are to be eaten raw without peeling (lettuce, for instance) and remove quite a thick layer of peel from carrots, cucumber, etc. There are specially designed products available for washing vegetables, or a little vinegar in the water will be a certain amount of help – but be sure to rinse thoroughly afterwards so that you do not give your candida a chance to enjoy the vinegar!

Taking a really good programme of appropriate vitamins and minerals will also help to protect you from the effects of pollutants, whether or not you are able to eat organic foods.

An important part of salads should be sprouted grains and beans, which provide protein as well as vitamins, minerals and fibre. These can be bought but it is so easy to grow your own from beans like aduki, mung beans, soybeans, alfalfa, chickpeas (garbanzos) and lentils (not split red lentils), and also from grains, especially wheat and barley. They each have their own flavour and can be used as lightly steamed vegetables as well as raw salad ingredients. It is possible to buy three-tier sprouters, but it is perfectly adequate to use a large jar with a muslin cover held in place by a rubber band. Take only enough beans or grains to allow them room in the jar to increase about eight times in bulk. This will probably be about three tablespoons in a two-pound jar. Cover the seeds with water and fix the muslin or a piece of nylon net over the top of the jar. Leave to soak overnight. In the morning, pour off the water then fill with fresh water and pour off again. Then lay the jar on its side. It does not have to be put in a dark cupboard; sprouting in the light appears to produce more vitamin C, so you can leave the jar on the kitchen windowsill. A warm spot is beneficial. For the next few days, rinse and drain the sprouts thoroughly two or three times daily. This is all you have to do, but do not leave any water in the jar or the seeds will rot. Bean sprouts may be eaten when the root is about 4cm/1½ inches long, but grain sprouts are best eaten when the root is about 12mm/½ inch. Sprouts may be kept in the refrigerator but still should be eaten within two days. They are best eaten as soon as they are ready.

Most root vegetables can be chopped or grated in a salad: carrots, turnips, parsnips, beetroot, radishes, mooli (which tastes like a mild radish), celeriac, fennel and, of course, spring onions (scallions). Finely sliced peppers – whether red, green or yellow – add flavour and are attractive, but avoid the very hot chilli peppers. And there are still those firm favourites, cucumber and tomato, without which no salad would be complete for many people!

Fresh herbs can bring delightful and unusual flavours to a bowl of salad, and bright orange marigold petals or pretty mauve chive heads can turn an ordinary green salad into something exotic.

Here are some interesting salad combinations to try:

- Sliced fennel with cauliflower florets and courgette (zucchini) cut into matchsticks.
- Celeriac and carrot cut into matchsticks with cauliflower florets.
- Carrot, beetroot and parsnip all cut into matchsticks.
- Sugar-snap peas, strips of yellow pepper and rings of radish.

Coleslaw

Coleslaw is a favourite with many people, but new 'yeasties' often think they cannot eat it because of the vinegar in the mayonnaise. A little further on you will find a recipe for vinegar-free mayonnaise which means you can still enjoy your coleslaw! However, there is just one word of warning about coleslaw. If you have been advised that you are suffering from an underactive thyroid (which quite often appears to be the case with sufferers from candida), it is a good idea to avoid raw cabbage because it actually inhibits the absorption of iodine, which is necessary for efficient thyroid activity. One of my clients had very low early-morning temperature readings, indicating that her thyroid was probably extremely underactive. I discovered that because she suffered from so many food allergies but could cope with raw cabbage, she had eaten it for lunch every single day for the past 11 years! For those whose thyroid is presenting no problems, here is a basic recipe for coleslaw:

---

* Coleslaw

GLUTEN-FREE

250g/8oz/4½ cups white cabbage, shredded
125g/4oz/¾ cup carrots, grated
3 spring onions (scallions), trimmed and chopped
Dressing *(pages 139–42)*

Mix all ingredients together.

If you need or wish to avoid raw white cabbage, it may be lightly steamed or cooked in a microwave and allowed to cool. Mixed with grated, crunchy raw carrot and a little onion it is quite acceptable as coleslaw. Don't try this with savoy or green cabbage, because they develop a rather strong smell and flavour.

Salad Dressings

Many people complain that they cannot manage to munch through a salad if it is dry. They seem to think that because they can no longer have salad cream from a jar, they have to do without. Let's have a look at some simple dressings.

Which oils are best? Olive oil tastes good in dressings, but is not the best nutritionally although it is the safest oil for cooking. Those which are most beneficial when taken cold include sunflower oil, safflower oil, sesame oil, linseed oil (flax) and rapeseed oil in an unrefined, cold-pressed form.

* Simple Dressing

GLUTEN-FREE

4 tbsp unrefined oil
4 tsp lemon juice, freshly squeezed
Optional: pinch of any dried herbs, or crushed garlic, or chopped chives, freshly ground
    black pepper

Stir ingredients together in a jug, or pour straight into bottom of salad bowl before adding salad ingredients, then 'toss' just before serving.

A larger quantity can be made in a screw-top jar and kept in the refrigerator for a few days, shaken well before use.

* Hummus Dressing

GLUTEN-FREE

If you have some home-made hummus ready (*see recipe in Chapter 14, page 106*), or have bought some fresh, just pile it on top of your salad for thick, garlic-flavoured dressing.

* Mayonnaise

1 free-range egg
2 tbsp fresh lemon juice
Optional: 5 tbsp of either chopped fresh tarragon or chives.
300ml/½ pint/1⅓ cups sunflower oil (or mixed sunflower and olive oils), unrefined
Pinch mustard powder
Freshly ground black pepper
1 tbsp boiling water

Beat the egg and lemon juice, using whisk or blender, till creamy. (If using herbs, stir in now.) Add the oil very gradually, beating continuously. Add the seasonings and lastly beat in the boiling water. Chill.

* Garlic Mayonnaise

Add 1 clove of garlic, crushed (or 1 tsp garlic granules) to the above recipe.

* Yoghurt Mayonnaise

150ml/¼ pint/⅔ cup mayonnaise, as above
150ml/¼ pint/⅔ cup natural yoghurt
Optional: ½ red pepper, finely chopped and/or 1 tsp paprika

Mix the mayonnaise and yoghurt. That's it – unless you're adding the chopped pepper and/or the paprika. Stir all together.

* Yoghurt Dressing 1

SIMPLEST OF ALL! – AND GLUTEN-FREE

Just use natural yoghurt as a dressing. It makes a really delicious coleslaw and couldn't be easier.

Optional: Add some finely chopped fresh mint or a sprinkling of dried mint.

* Yoghurt Dressing 2

GLUTEN-FREE

270ml/8fl oz/1 cup natural yoghurt
1 onion, finely chopped
½ clove garlic, crushed
Juice of half a lemon
Freshly ground black pepper

Mix ingredients by hand or in a processor.

* Yoghurt Dressing 3

GLUTEN-FREE

230ml/8fl oz/1 cup natural yoghurt
½ cup unrefined oil (see notes on page 50)
Juice of half a lemon
2 tbsp chives, finely chopped
2 tbsp parsley, finely chopped
1 clove garlic, crushed
½ tsp mustard powder
Freshly ground black pepper

Blend in a processor or liquidizer till smooth. Chill.

* Tofu and Lemon Dressing

GLUTEN-FREE

1 packet tofu
2 tbsp fresh lemon juice
2 tbsp unrefined oil *(see notes on page 50)*
1 clove garlic, crushed (or ½ tsp garlic granules)

Blend in a processor or liquidizer until smooth. Chill.

Buffet Salads

So far I have only discussed variations on raw salad vegetables, but a salad buffet table can look so attractive and appetizing if there are bowls of other types of salad as well. The following are a few ideas:

* Chickpeas (Garbanzos) in Tomato Dressing

GLUTEN-FREE

1 can chickpeas (garbanzos), or 225g/8oz/1⅓ cups home-cooked chickpeas (garbanzos)
4 tbsp finely chopped onion
2 tbsp chopped parsley
2 tbsp chopped fresh herbs
2 cloves of garlic, crushed
6 tbsp unrefined sunflower oil
2 tbsp freshly-squeezed lemon juice
4 tbsp tomato purée (no citric acid)

Put chickpeas (garbanzos) into a bowl. Mix together the ingredients for the dressing, add to chickpeas (garbanzos) and stir thoroughly. Served with a green salad and whole-grain rice, this makes a very nutritious meal.

* Chickpea (Garbanzo) or Beany Salad

GLUTEN-FREE

2 sticks of celery
½ green pepper
1 medium tomato
2 spring onions (scallions), or 1 small purple onion
75g/3oz/½ cup cucumber
½ can sweetcorn, drained and rinsed
1 can chickpeas (garbanzos) or any mixture of beans, drained and rinsed

Wash and finely chop celery, green pepper, tomato, onions and cucumber (peeled). Mix all ingredients together and toss with any of the previous dressings or with natural yoghurt.

* Pasta Salad

MAY BE GLUTEN-FREE

175g/6oz/2 cups uncooked wholemeal macaroni or other pasta shapes (gluten-free pasta
    may be used – rice, corn, buckwheat)
125g/4oz/1 cup prawns
1 carrot
3 spring onions (scallions)
1 yellow or red pepper
1 stick of celery
1 tomato
A few radishes

Cook macaroni or other pasta shapes and allow to cool. If using frozen prawns, allow to defrost. Wash, peel and chop all vegetables. Mix all ingredients together and toss with a yoghurt dressing.

* Potato Salad

225g/½lb/1½ cups new potatoes
2 free-range eggs
2 spring onions (scallions)
4 radishes
2 sticks of celery
1 carrot

Thoroughly wash and scrub new potatoes, boil with their skins on, allow to cool and then cut into cubes. Hard-boil (10 minutes) the eggs, then crack their shells and cool under running water (to prevent discoloration). Take off the shells, allow eggs to finish cooling, then chop into small pieces. Wash and peel the vegetables, as appropriate, then chop the onions, radishes and celery and grate the carrot. Mix all ingredients together and toss with a yoghurt dressing or yoghurt mayonnaise.

Chapter 19

Sauces and Stuffings

When people first start on the anti-candida diet, they often complain that the food tastes bland and uninteresting. There are several reasons for this. First, if you are deficient in zinc, this will affect your senses of taste and smell, so after a few weeks on a good supplement programme you will start to find that food has considerably more flavour than you realized. In addition, both salt and sugar have the effect of 'anaesthetizing' the taste buds. One friend, having overcome candida, experimented gently with some honey in a recipe – and found that for the rest of that day her food had no flavour!

Having said all of this, there really is no need to think that anti-candida food is tasteless, and a good savoury sauce can do a great deal to make your meal more interesting.

---

* Basic 'White' Sauce

GLUTEN-FREE IF USING FINE MAIZE MEAL OR RICE FLOUR

I put the inverted commas in the title because it is impossible, using unrefined grains, to make a conventional sauce which is as white as one made with refined white flour or cornflour (cornstarch).

25g/1oz/large knob unsalted butter
2 tbsp fine maize meal (or brown rice flour or wholemeal flour)
300ml/½ pint/1⅓ cups soya milk (or rice milk)

Optional: freshly ground black pepper, softened chopped onion, bay leaf, mace, mixed herbs, chopped parsley, chopped chives, etc.

Melt the butter in a saucepan over a low heat. Remove pan from heat and add the flour, mixing to a smooth paste. Gradually add soya milk, stirring all the time. Bring to the boil, stirring, reduce heat and simmer for 2 minutes. The result should be a smooth paste, which you can flavour and season as required.

---

* Fat-free White Sauce

This can be made by excluding butter from the previous recipe. Make a paste with the flour (whichever type you prefer) and some of the soya milk. Stir over low heat, gradually add the rest of the soya milk and bring to the boil, stirring constantly. Flavour as desired.

** Tomato and Onion Sauce 1

GLUTEN-FREE

1 small onion
Optional: 1 clove garlic
1 tbsp extra virgin olive oil
400g/14oz can tomatoes (no citric acid)
2 tsp brown rice flour
½ lemon, squeezed

Chop onion and garlic. Put in a pan with the oil over moderate heat to soften but not brown. Add tomatoes but reserve the juice. Lightly mash tomatoes into the onions and heat through for about 5 minutes. Mix flour with the lemon juice and reserved tomato juice and add carefully, stirring all the time, and cook for about 3 minutes.

** Tomato and Onion Sauce 2

GLUTEN-FREE IF USING RICE FLOUR

1 medium onion
2 tomatoes, skinned and cored
1 tbsp extra virgin olive oil
1 tbsp tomato purée (no citric acid)
1 tsp wholewheat flour (or brown rice flour)
Freshly ground black pepper
Pinch of mixed herbs
150ml/¼ pint/⅔ cup vegetable stock

Sauté onion and tomatoes in oil for 5 minutes. Add tomato purée, flour, pepper, herbs and stock, stirring well. Simmer for 5 minutes, stirring frequently.

* Easiest Tomato and Onion Sauce 3

GLUTEN-FREE

1 medium onion
1 tbsp extra virgin olive oil
1 can tomatoes (no citric acid)
Optional: pinch of oregano or mixed herbs or 1 tbsp tomato purée for extra richness

Chop onion and soften in the oil (up to 4 minutes in saucepan or microwave). Add can of tomatoes roughly mashed, together with optional flavourings, then heat through.

* Fat-free Tomato and Onion Sauce 4

GLUTEN-FREE

2 tsp tomato purée (no citric acid)
150ml/¼ pint/⅔ cup vegetable stock or filtered water
1 medium onion, chopped

Optional: bay leaf, freshly ground black pepper, pinch cumin, coriander, turmeric, mixed
    spices, oregano
Optional: 2 tsp fine maize meal, canned tomatoes (no citric acid)

Mix the purée with the liquid. Add the onion, and soften by cooking over a moderate
heat for a few minutes. Flavour as required. This may be used just as it is with a small
can of tuna, for instance, or thickened by adding maize meal (stirred in carefully over a
low heat and brought briefly to the boil) or some tomatoes from a can.

** Tomato-less Pasta Sauce

GLUTEN-FREE, SERVES 2–3

Many sauces contain tomato, which is difficult if you happen to have an intolerance to
this useful member of the nightshade family. Nevertheless, it is not impossible to make
a really tasty sauce without tomatoes.

For a fast, fat-free version of this pasta sauce, steam all the vegetables instead of
baking or sautéing, although the red pepper may still be grilled.

2 red peppers
½ butternut squash
2 courgettes (zucchini)
1–2 tbsp extra virgin olive oil
2 leeks (or 1 onion)
Vegetable stock
½ tsp mixed herbs

Wash, halve and de-seed the red peppers. Place cut side down under a hot grill until
skins are dark. Leave to cool. Peel (or scoop out) the butternut and dice the flesh. Wash
and slice courgettes (zucchini). Put courgettes (zucchini) and butternut into a baking
dish, thinly coat with some of the olive oil and bake for 45 minutes at 375°F/190°C/Gas
Mark 5. Slice and sauté the leeks or onion gently in a frying pan with the remaining olive
oil until softened. Skin and dice the red peppers. Mix all vegetables together, then put
half of them into a liquidizer and blend with sufficient vegetable stock to give the consistency of a thick soup. Return to saucepan and add the rest of the vegetables, stirring in
mixed herbs, and reheat. Serve with the pasta of your choice, and possibly increase the
protein content by adding a can of chickpeas (garbanzos) or other beans.

---

* Chicken and Lemon Sauce

GLUTEN-FREE

Juices from a roasted chicken
½ lemon, squeezed
½ small carton Greek yoghurt

Strain the fat off the chicken juices, add the lemon juice and yoghurt. Serve with chicken. (N.B. You can cook the chicken with the lemon juice poured over it and the squeezed lemon shell inside the breast cavity, in which case you just add the yoghurt to the chicken juices – see recipe for Lemon Bay Chicken, *page 188.*)

** Tomato Ketchup

GLUTEN-FREE

1 large onion
1 tbsp extra virgin olive oil
225g/½lb/1⅓ cups tomatoes
1 clove garlic
1 bay leaf
Pinch of dried basil, oregano and rosemary (or 1 tsp each, if fresh, and finely chopped)
1 tbsp fresh parsley, finely chopped

Finely chop the onion, add to oil and heat gently till soft. Chop the tomatoes and garlic and add to onions together with bay leaf and herbs. Stir. Cook over low heat until tomatoes are very soft. Remove bay leaf. Mash the sauce well or purée in a blender. Allow to cool, put in an airtight jar in the refrigerator for a short time, or freeze in yoghurt tubs till needed.

** Bread Sauce 1

GLUTEN-FREE BREAD MAY BE USED, *SEE PAGES 76–7*

This makes a traditional bread sauce to serve with turkey. You need to start it well in advance.

1 medium onion
12 cloves
425ml/¾ pint/2 cups soya milk (or rice milk)
1 bay leaf
6 black peppercorns
75g/3oz/1⅓ cups freshly made breadcrumbs from yeast-free wholemeal soda bread *(see pages 72–8)*
50g/2oz/¼ cup unsalted butter (or 2 tbsp unrefined sunflower oil)

Cut the onion in half and stick cloves into it, then put it in a saucepan with the soya milk, bay leaf and peppercorns and leave for 2 hours in a warm place – standing by or on the cooker where the turkey is cooking, for instance. Then bring the milk to the boil as slowly as possible. Remove but keep the onion, bay leaf and peppercorns.

Meanwhile, make the breadcrumbs (a liquidizer is helpful) and stir them into the boiled milk with half the butter. Put the saucepan over a very low heat and stir occasionally, until the bread has swollen. Replace the onion with its cloves and the bay leaf, and put the sauce back in its warm place till needed. Heat through at the last moment, remove onion and bay leaf, beat in the remaining butter and serve hot.

* Bread Sauce 2

GLUTEN-FREE IF USING QUINOA

This can also be used as a replacement for potatoes or rice at a main meal, in which case you could use your favourite herbs to add flavour, though lovage is particularly recommended.

125g/4oz/¾ cup quinoa (or bulgar)
450ml/¾ pint/2 cups boiling water
1 yeast-free soya stock cube

1 onion (or 4 shallots), finely sliced
1 tsp extra virgin olive oil
1 bay leaf
3 cloves
Freshly ground black pepper

Wash quinoa or bulgar thoroughly in a fine sieve. Put all ingredients in a saucepan and bring to the boil. Simmer on low heat for 10–12 minutes, until dry.

* Millet Stuffing

GLUTEN-FREE

170g/6oz/1 cup millet
1 tbsp extra virgin olive oil
1 small onion (or 2 shallots)
3 cups water and 1 stock cube (or 3 cups stock)
Optional: crushed garlic, marjoram, oregano, pepper, bay leaf, etc.

Wash millet in fine sieve and drain carefully in kitchen paper. Heat oil in wok or frying pan and add millet. Gently brown for a few minutes and add finely sliced onion or shallots, stirring until slightly brown in places. Turn into good-sized saucepan. Bring stock to the boil, add herbs if using, pour onto millet, cover and simmer until stock is absorbed – about 25 minutes. Use to stuff chicken or turkey, or put into a roasting tin to brown in the oven (20–30 minutes at 350°F/180°C/Gas Mark 4) and then serve separately. Alternatively, make into small balls before browning in the oven.

* Wheatgerm Stuffing

4 heaped tbsp wheatgerm
2 tbsp chopped parsley
1 tsp mixed dried herbs
freshly grated nutmeg, to taste

freshly ground black pepper
1 small onion, finely chopped
1 tbsp olive oil
1 egg yolk
1 tsp lemon juice, freshly squeezed
water to mix

Mix dry ingredients in a bowl, then thoroughly mix in the rest. Add sufficient water to make a stiff dropping consistency. Put into chicken or turkey before roasting (remember to add the weight of the stuffing to the weight of the bird when calculating time), or bake separately in an oiled roasting tin, 20–30 minutes at 350°F/190°C/Gas Mark 5.

* Traditional Sage and Onion Stuffing

GLUTEN-FREE IF USING CORN BREAD

2 onions, finely chopped
2 tsp dried sage (or 2 tbsp chopped fresh sage)
1½ mugs soda breadcrumbs (see page 73) or corn breadcrumbs (see page 76)
½ tsp paprika
Freshly ground black pepper

Preheat oven to 375°F/190°C/Gas Mark 5. Cover the onions with water in a pan, add the sage and bring to the boil. Simmer gently until onion is soft and water has reduced to 3–4 tbsp. Stir in the breadcrumbs, paprika and a shake of black pepper. Make into little balls and bake in oven at the same time as the chicken, using bottom shelf.

*** Rice and Chestnut Stuffing

GLUTEN-FREE

Preparing the chestnuts is time-consuming, but in our family it is regularly part of the anticipation and excitement in the countdown days to Christmas, though I have to confess that this is a job where Daddy (now Grandpa) takes over!

900g/2lb/5 cups chestnuts in their shells (or frozen)
225g/½lb/1 cup long-grain brown rice
1 free-range egg
1 tbsp extra virgin olive oil
2 tbsp chopped parsley
Optional: freshly ground black pepper

Cut a cross in each of the chestnuts, so they will not explode, then put them in a large pan of boiling water for about five minutes. Handle them as hot as possible, and you will find that the shell and inner skin come away quite easily, using a sharp knife. Of course, frozen de-shelled chestnuts save a lot of time and effort, and they do taste pretty good.

Boil the shelled nuts for about 5 minutes if you like a nutty consistency, 10 minutes if you like the stuffing to be softer. Chop them roughly. Boil the rice in double the quantity of water, until all the water has been absorbed (30–40 minutes). In a large bowl, mix the chopped chestnuts with the rice and also mix in the egg, oil and parsley, with some freshly ground black pepper if required. Stuff the body cavity of the turkey, and allow an extra 1½ kg/3lb to the weight of the bird when calculating cooking times. Alternatively, bake the stuffing separately in an oiled roasting tin for 30 minutes, if there's room in the oven with the turkey!

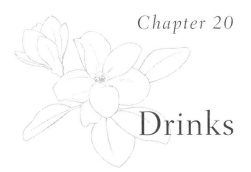

Chapter 20

Drinks

More often than not, one of the first hurdles which needs to be jumped is coming off tea and coffee. It is quite amazing just how much these highly socially-acceptable drinks are damaging the health of the civilized world. I have seen complete personality changes within a few days of tea and coffee being stopped. Depression, anxiety, insomnia, irritability and a whole range of physical symptoms can sometimes vanish into thin air within a week of breaking an unsuspected addiction to the stimulants contained in them – which are just as addictive as heroin. The immune system reacts to these stimulants as it would to a foreign invader and, in order to keep the symptoms at bay, we need to keep taking these stimulants by drinking more tea and coffee. However, if we want to build up the immune system so that it can better cope with fighting off candida, we need to remove this burden on the adrenal glands which has been weakening our immunity.

Another problem with any food or drink which acts as a stimulant is that it provokes the adrenal glands to trigger the release of the body's sugar stores (as does stress of any sort), and this surge of sugar into the bloodstream gives candida a beanfeast.

So, it really is essential to get tea and coffee (and also chocolate and cola drinks, which contain some of the same stimulants) out of our lives and out of our systems. When you first give them up, you can expect to have quite a severe headache because you will be experiencing symptoms of drug-withdrawal. Most people get over this in a couple of days, so you need to choose a time when you haven't got much to do, perhaps a weekend. It is no good trying to wean yourself off these stimulants; being addicted to them means that you will simply want more all the time. You need to find an alternative drink which you quite enjoy and then just make up your mind to go for it. (For further discussion of tea and coffee, *see below*.)

What alternatives are there? Well, first there is the whole range of herbal teas and fruit teas. Although fruit itself (and fruit juices) are not allowed, the majority of fruit teas are fine because they contain hardly any fructose, but you do need to read the labels carefully because sometimes they contain added malt or citric acid. Don't automatically assume that a supermarket brand of fruit tea is 'safe'; quite often they contain unhelpful substances such as unnatural flavouring, so read the labels very carefully. There is plenty of variety and choice from reputable companies on sale in health-food stores.

Many people find rooibosch (red bush) the closest to 'proper' tea, and are surprised to find that they like it. A good alternative to coffee is Barleycup because it has a roasted flavour, but it is made from barley, rye and chicory. You might miss the smell of coffee to start with, but the smell of roasted grains will grow on you! It makes a pleasant hot drink, either black or with soya milk or rice milk. There are several similar drinks available but they usually contain a sweetening agent such as malt, figs or dates, so again you must be careful to read the labels.

Dandelion coffee, made from dandelion root, is another good coffee-substitute but the instant variety, available in jars, contains lactose so must be avoided. Instead, you can buy roasted dandelion root in packets. See the following recipes for how to make it. Dandelion root is extremely good for you because it helps to clean up the liver by stimulating the production of bile, the substance which carries toxins out with it. People experiencing die-off symptoms would benefit by drinking lots of dandelion root coffee; in fact it is so pleasant that you could well make it your regular hot drink during the day.

How much fluid to drink is discussed in Chapter 7, but in fact the more you have the better, especially when your body needs to eliminate toxins. Filter jugs for water are definitely a good idea, and there are also companies who will plumb in a water-filter system to your kitchen sink, or else supply a free-standing table-top model which looks quite attractive and provides water with a superb quality and flavour. It's certainly worth considering if you have cause to be concerned about the pollution factor in your health equation.

A glass of sparkling water with a slice of lemon when you are out for an evening makes a refreshing and socially-acceptable drink. If you are worried about what your friends in the bar might think, who's to know it doesn't contain some vodka?! At home, you might like to put some fizz in your water occasionally by using a soda siphon. And here's a tip I picked up in Belfast – besides adding a slice of well-scrubbed lemon, add a slice of cucumber. Delicious!

The point about sociability is important. Clients are sometimes more worried about what other people will think than about the fact that they are giving up their favourite alcoholic drink, although candida can actually cause an addiction to alcohol, especially beer or wine which are high in yeast. The problem is that if you break your diet because of either real or imagined social pressure, *you* are the one who will suffer the consequences, not your friends. You will encourage some additional candida activity and then this will be followed by additional die-off reaction. Is it really worth it?

Hot drinks when you are out and about present no problem if you use a little forethought and always carry some herbal teabags or a little empty pill-pot filled with Barleycup in your handbag or pocket. Any restaurant or friend will gladly supply you with a cup or jug of hot water, and you can quietly make your own drink. It may provoke some interest, but that just gives you a good opportunity to tell people how much better you feel for not drinking tea or coffee, and it may be the first step towards helping someone else. We tend to think that no one else has problems because everyone goes around looking pretty normal; you will find there are very few who are not coping with health problems to some extent and would be better for a change in diet.

Apart from the wide range of different flavours of herb teas which are available, you can have fun making some of your own. You can make any flavoured tea using fresh or dried herbs by following these simple directions – a good reason for growing your own herbs, many of which have very pretty flowers and look attractive in the garden. Even packaged herb teas like rooibosch can be given an extra zing by adding a couple of fresh mint leaves.

---

* Mint Tea

15g/½oz/1 cup of mint leaves, chopped (or 7g/¼oz/½ cup dried mint leaves)
1.2 litres/2 pints/5 cups boiling water

Cover the mint with the water and leave overnight. Strain and reheat.

OR put mint and water into a saucepan, bring to the boil, cover and simmer for 20 minutes.

---

* Cinnamon Tea

2 sticks of cinnamon
½ organic lemon, scrubbed, grated and squeezed
425ml/15fl oz/2 cups water

Put the cinnamon, lemon juice, lemon peel and water into a saucepan, bring to the boil, cover and simmer for 20 minutes.

* Iced Teas

Herb teas and fruit teas (made extra strong) can also be drunk cold or iced in the summer, and make a refreshing change from water. Put some ice cubes into an attractive glass jug, pour the cold herb tea over it, and add some slices of lemon or mint leaves. If you like, the jug could be half-filled with chilled herb or fruit tea and topped up with sparkling mineral water. Could anyone possibly prefer orange squash from a bottle?

* Sparkling Yoghurt Drink

For a cold drink with a difference – a sort of alternative to milk shake – try this sparkling yoghurt drink.

1 small carton natural yoghurt
Sparking mineral water
Optional: 1–2 drops natural vanilla essence
Fresh mint to garnish

Whisk the yoghurt until frothy and mix with sparkling mineral water – how much depends on whether you prefer a drink which is thick and creamy or one which is rather lighter. Add some natural vanilla essence, serve it with a straw, and you have a popular drink which will encourage yeasty children to take more yoghurt, and therefore more calcium. Grown-ups can have it, too!

* Dandelion Root Coffee

GLUTEN-FREE

2 heaped tsp roasted dandelion root
2 litres/3½ pints/9 cups filtered water

Place dandelion root pieces in a saucepan with the water, bring to the boil, reduce heat and simmer for 15 minutes. Strain. Reheat a cupful when required.

Alternatively, if you have a grinder and coffee-making equipment (filter jug, percolator, coffee machine), grind the root pieces and proceed as if you were making proper coffee. (N.B. Do not use like instant coffee.)

* Winter Warmer

1 piece ginger root (preferably organic)
1 piece liquorice root
6 black peppercorns
1 piece cinnamon stick
2 spice cloves
575ml/1 pint/2½ cups filtered water

Peel and grate the ginger root and squeeze pulp into a cup to express the juice – about 6 drops is enough. Place all ingredients into a small pan with the water and simmer gently for 15 minutes. Drink hot. This client says she drinks it to warm herself up before she goes out, and another cup of it to wrap her numb fingers around when she comes back home. She also finds it marvellously soothing to sip if she has a sore throat. And if you use *organic* ginger root, she says the flavour is something else!

* Christmas Fruit and Spice Hot Punch

Who needs wine or spirits? You can keep going all over the festive season on this delicious punch without worrying about candida or your liver!

Ingredients of Winter Warmer recipe, plus
5 teabags rosehip and hibiscus

Prepare Winter Warmer ingredients as in previous recipe but don't add the water. Make fruit tea by boiling the water and pouring over teabags in a heatproof jug. Allow to infuse until cool. Squeeze the bags before removing, then pour fruit tea into a saucepan with the Winter Warmer ingredients for 15 minutes. Allow to cool slightly before pouring a measure into a glass.

* Cappuccino

You don't even have to miss out on Cappuccino!

1 cup soya milk (choose a 'creamy' variety)
1 tsp Barleycup (or roasted chicory powder)
A little carob powder

Boil the soya milk, adding Barleycup or chicory powder and stirring well. When boiled, whisk and pour into a mug. Sprinkle with a little carob powder. (N.B. Rice milk does not froth up as well as soya milk.)

Chapter 21

Rice and Other Grains

When using any grains, you should buy only whole grains. This means that the only part which has been removed is the husk, which is indigestible. When grains are refined, the outer layers are removed and many valuable nutrients are lost, whereas the whole grain provides excellent nourishment and fibre. Rice is probably the grain which is most commonly used as part of a main meal, so let's look at different ways of cooking it.

---

* Whole-Grain Rice

GLUTEN-FREE

Allow one cup of rice for two people (or use a mug if you have big appetites). Put into a saucepan, and for each cup of rice add two cups of filtered water. Bring to the boil then reduce heat so that the water is barely simmering. Cover with a tight lid and cook for 30–40 minutes. All the water will be absorbed and the grains will remain separate. (Check towards the end of the time in case you need to add a little more boiling water.)

Rice cooks well in a microwave oven. Allow the same quantities and cook in a deep covered casserole dish on High for about 30 minutes.

Rice cooked in stock instead of water will have a savoury flavour. Or you can add ½ teaspoon of turmeric to give flavour and an attractive yellow colour. Chopped onion, chopped fresh parsley or a variety of herbs and spices can also be added during cooking, so rice need never be thought of as 'plain and boring'. Try a bay leaf, or cumin and coriander – depending on what is to be eaten with the rice.

Whole-grain basmati rice gives a delicious variation. Cook it in the same way. Alternatives to rice are wheat berries and forms of cracked or ground wheat called couscous and bulgar (which has been partly pre-cooked). Then there is millet, pot barley (not pearl barley, which is polished), buckwheat and rye groats. If you have found that your body cannot tolerate gluten, you need to avoid wheat, rye, oats and barley, but you can still enjoy rice, maize (corn), millet, buckwheat and quinoa. Quinoa is fairly new to our shops and is highly nutritious, being very rich in protein. Look out for it, and try it in a pilaff, using the Bread Sauce 2 recipe on page 150. Let's look at ways of cooking these various grains.

* Quinoa

GLUTEN-FREE

This has an interesting, nutty flavour.

Bring 225g/8oz of quinoa to the boil in 900ml/1½ pints/3¾ cups of water. Simmer on a low heat for 10–12 minutes, until dry.

* Wheat Berries

Wheat berries are the whole grain of the wheat. When cooked they make a delicious, slightly chewy alternative to rice. They are excellent served cold in salads.

Take 225g/8oz wheat berries, cover in boiling water and soak for 1 hour. Drain and cover with 900ml/1½ pints/3¾ cups boiling water. Cover with a tight lid and simmer for 1 hour, replenishing water if necessary.

Microwave: cover with boiling water, quantities as above, then cook on High for 30 minutes, allow to stand for 20 minutes, and drain.

* Bulgar Wheat

Put 1 cup of bulgar wheat into a saucepan with 2 cups of water. Bring to the boil, cover, and simmer over a very low heat for 15 minutes.

Alternatively, pour boiling water onto the bulgar, cover and leave to stand for 30 minutes; couldn't be easier!

Microwave: cover with boiling water, quantities as above, then cook on High for 2–3 minutes, and allow to stand for 5 minutes.

* Couscous

Cook the same way as bulgar.

* Millet

GLUTEN-FREE

This grain has more flavour if it is gently cooked in a pan with a little olive oil for a few minutes before boiling. Then bring it to the boil in twice the quantity of water, cover with a tight lid and simmer for at least 30 minutes, until fluffy.

Microwave: cover with boiling water, quantities as above, cook on High for 15 minutes and allow to stand for 4 minutes.

* Pot Barley

Soak and cook as for wheat berries, allowing at least 1 hour.

* Roasted Buckwheat

GLUTEN-FREE

Cook as for rice, allowing 20–30 minutes.

* Rye Groats

Soak and cook as for wheat berries.

Serve any of these grains with a hot meal, making healthy and filling alternatives to potato or pasta. They can be served in a 'dry' dish, like kedgeree or pilaff, or they can be used with a savoury hot sauce, or they can simply be an enjoyable way of soaking up the gravy from a chicken casserole or bean stew. If you have some left over, try mixing it next day with beans and chopped-up raw vegetables to make an interesting salad.

* Tabbouleh

This interesting grain salad from the Middle East uses bulgar wheat and is therefore very easy to make.

170g/6oz/1 cup bulgar wheat
425ml/15fl oz/2 cups boiling water
4 tbsp chopped spring onions (scallions)
4 tbsp chopped fresh parsley
2 tbsp chopped green pepper
510g/18oz/3 cups chopped tomato
345g/12oz/3 cups chopped celery
2 tbsp chopped fresh mint
4 tbsp unrefined sunflower oil or extra virgin olive oil
Juice of 1 lemon

Soak the bulgar in the boiling water for 30 minutes. Drain to make sure it is completely dry. Mix all ingredients together, omitting any not to hand and adding any others such as cucumber. Experiment and have fun!

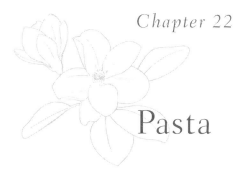

Chapter 22

Pasta

This chapter will not contain actual recipes for using pasta as these appear in other chapters, such as Chapter 23 'Pulses and Seeds', Chapter 24 'Meat and Poultry' and Chapter 25 'Fish'. All I intend to do here is make you aware of the fact that there is plenty of wholewheat pasta available in the shops, even in many ordinary supermarkets, and obviously it makes a good accompaniment or basis for many main meals. Some clients do need to be told this, because they look at the diet sheet and feel at first that there is absolutely nothing in the world they can eat!

Unless the packet specifically claims that the contents are made from wholewheat, you should not buy it. For instance, *pasta verde* is coloured with spinach to make it green, but the wheat used will be refined unless the packet actually says it is wholewheat, which it usually does not.

There are many different types of pasta – spaghetti, shells, spirals and lasagne. It is even possible to buy pre-cooked wholewheat lasagne, which makes the job much easier and cuts down the cooking time. Make up your sauce and then use the pre-cooked lasagne according to the directions on the packet. Other types of pasta simply need putting into a large pan of boiling water for 10–12 minutes and draining. Wholewheat seems to need a little longer than the refined variety. However, don't let it overcook or you will end up with a sticky, soggy mass! For a real Italian touch, stir a little olive oil into the pasta before serving. Use it with any savoury dish you fancy. For quantity, you should allow 150–175g (5–6oz/1¾–2 cups) of pasta (that means its dry, pre-cooked weight) per person, or more depending on appetite.

You can sometimes find buckwheat spaghetti, which is fine for a gluten-free diet, but some makes also contain wheat, so check the label. Other useful forms of gluten-free pasta are spaghetti and shells made from maize (unrefined corn) and from whole rice. Small children love the little shells, which make an appetizing and nutritious meal with a bean and vegetable sauce *(see pages 169–70)*.

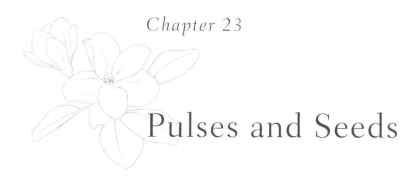

Chapter 23

Pulses and Seeds

'Pulse' is simply the name given to any kind of pea, bean or lentil. In this chapter I am discussing dried pulses, which are extremely nutritious and, if eaten with a whole grain as in wholewheat pasta, pastry or brown rice, combine to give a 'complete' protein – far more cheaply than meat and without the saturated fat content, which is very high even in lean meat.

I was delighted that far more recipes came in from my clients for this chapter than for any other, showing that many of them had learned the pleasure and economic sense of eating this type of food.

You can have a lot of fun creating meals with pulses. First there are all the different types (which we will look at in a moment), then there are the different flavoured sauces you can use with them – onion, tomato, parsley, herb, lemon, spicy – and then there are all the different ways of using them – pies, pasties, crumbles, lasagnes, bologneses, pancakes, risottos, paellas, quiches and burgers.

Cooking Pulses

Most beans need to be soaked overnight before cooking (I will point out those which don't). You usually do this simply in cold water, but in the case of chickpeas (garbanzos), kidney beans (red or white) and soya beans, you should boil them for at least 10 minutes before leaving them to soak in the hot water. After soaking, always drain and rinse the beans and cover them with fresh cold water for cooking. Bring to the boil again, lower the heat and simmer till tender (*see times to allow on pages 167–9*).

If you have forgotten to soak the beans overnight, you can bring them slowly to the boil in a large pan of water, boil for at least 10 minutes then leave them to soak in the hot water for an hour. Drain and rinse, cover with cold water and bring to the boil again, then turn down the heat and simmer till tender. You can tell if beans are ready by taking some out with a spoon and blowing on them to see if the skins burst open. Don't put them back in the pot!

If you take the precaution of changing the rinsing water before cooking, and then rinsing again *after* cooking (by putting them into a colander held over the sink and pouring boiling water over them), you will be far less likely to suffer from the dreaded 'wind' so associated with eating beans! It's the gluey substance that clings to them which is largely responsible.

If you use a pressure cooker, you can cut the cooking time by half. It's a good idea to cook lots of beans at a time, then freeze them in 125g/4oz or 225g/8oz packs.

Types of Pulse

Aduki Beans

Small, reddish-brown beans. They are just about small enough to get away with cooking in a reasonable length of time, about one hour, without pre-soaking. However, if you have time, soak for a few hours and then cook for 30–40 minutes. Good with brown rice.

Black-eyed Beans

White beans with a black spot. Soak overnight then cook for 40 minutes. Good cold in mixed salads.

Butter Beans

Large white beans. Good liquidized in stock for thick soup, or mashed into a bean pâté. Soak overnight then cook for one hour.

Field Beans

Round, brown beans. Soak overnight then cook for 30 minutes.

Flageolets

Small haricot bean, picked while still green. Soak overnight then cook for 45–60 minutes. Interesting, delicate flavour.

Haricot Beans

Kidney-shaped white beans, smaller than butter beans. Soak overnight then cook for one hour. Useful for making your own equivalent of beans in tomato sauce (*see 'Quick Home-made Baked Beans', page 175*).

Kidney Beans – Red or White

Essential to boil for 10 minutes before soaking overnight, then cook for one hour. Red kidney beans are used to make chilli con carne, and although a yeasty person should avoid such hot dishes, you can make an equivalent dish using gentler spices like cumin and coriander.

Soya Beans

Usually yellow and round, though there are different types. They contain all eight essential amino acids, so they provide as much protein as fillet steak! However, they are very hard, so after boiling for 10 minutes and a good long overnight soak they should be cooked for 3–4 hours. They have a lovely creamy texture, good for blending for pâtés. If using a pressure cooker, add 1 tablespoon of lemon juice; this stops the water frothing up. Cooking at pressure for 30 minutes should be adequate.

Green Lentils

No need to soak. Rinse and pick over for small stones. Put in a saucepan and add plenty of boiling water. Simmer for 45 minutes.

Red Split Lentils

These become mushy very quickly and are useful for thickening soups and stews. No need to soak. Rinse and pick over for small stones. Add to stock and cook for 15 minutes.

Brown Lentils

(Sometimes known as Continental lentils.) No need to soak. Rinse and pick over for small stones. Put in a saucepan and add plenty of boiling water. Simmer for 45–60 minutes. Use instead of minced beef for spaghetti bolognese, in a delicious sauce of tomatoes, onions and oregano, and I defy anyone who is prejudiced against vegetarian foods to realize that they are not eating minced beef! You can tell them as soon as they have said how much they enjoyed it.

Beware – all lentils should be well washed and sorted because they often have tiny stones in with them.

Chickpeas (Garbanzos)

A creamy-coloured legume that looks like a round nut. Boil for 10 minutes before leaving to soak overnight in the hot water, then cook for 2–3 hours. Good in a vegetable pie, or with rice, or liquidized to make hummus.

Whole Dried Peas

Soak overnight then cook for 45 minutes. Use whole as an accompaniment or mashed to make pease pudding.

Split Peas – Green or Yellow

No need to soak. Cooking time varies depending on whether you want them whole or mushy, about 30–40 minutes. Add to stock and cook for 40 minutes and you have lovely thick broth.

Bean Dishes

Having received so many recipes for beans, choosing just a few has been quite difficult. I have tried to use those which work on the principle that a pulse and grain together make a complete protein. Sometimes I have combined several ideas to make just one recipe; for instance, there are many different ways of making a bean and vegetable stew or casserole and, having made it, you can serve it with a large baked potato or with brown rice, in a lasagne or with pasta shells, with pastry over and under it to make a pie that will slice, with crumble topping on top and served with a side-salad, with dumplings in it for a warming stew, or you can put little scones on top and call it a cobbler ... the possibilities are endless, all from one basic recipe. So here it is.

*** (**) Bean and Vegetable Stew

GLUTEN-FREE BUT CAN BE SERVED WITH A GRAIN

Although specific measurements and types of beans and vegetables are given in this recipe, remember that it really doesn't matter what you use, and it can have as few or as many types of vegetable as you like. You can save your energy by using frozen vegetables and canned beans. Wash all fresh vegetables well.

4 tbsp extra virgin olive oil

1 large onion (or 2 medium onions), chopped

4 tsp fresh herbs (or 1 tsp dried herbs)

4 bay leaves

4 medium carrots, scrubbed and sliced

4 sticks celery, cut into 2.5cm/1-inch slices

1 small turnip, peeled and diced

1 small swede, peeled and diced

1 small parsnip, peeled and sliced

125g/4oz/⅔ cup fresh or frozen broad beans

1 green pepper, seeded and chopped

125g/4oz/1 cup cauliflower florets

250g/½lb/1½ cups tomatoes, chopped

4 tbsp tomato purée (no citric acid)

Water to cover

375g/12oz/1¾ cups (uncooked weight) haricot beans or (2¼ cups) kidney beans or (1¾ cups) chickpeas (garbanzos) soaked overnight then cooked (*see pages 167–9*) OR

2 large cans of beans (no sugar), drained and well rinsed

1 clove garlic, crushed

4 tbsp chopped parsley

Freshly ground black pepper

Pour the oil into a large saucepan or pressure cooker. Add the onion, herbs and bay leaves and cook over a low heat for 5 minutes. Add the carrot, celery, turnip, swede, parsnip, broad beans, pepper, cauliflower, tomatoes, tomato purée and enough water to just cover, and cook gently until the vegetables are tender, 5–10 minutes according to preference. Add the cooked beans, garlic, parsley and pepper. This makes enough to serve a hungry family, or you can eat some and freeze the rest in useful sized containers, or you can make it up into pieces to freeze, or liquidize some and put into pasties.

* Bean and Vegetable Stew – Simple Version

2 medium onions, chopped

1 green pepper, seeded and chopped

4 large cups of any other vegetables, chopped

Erica White's Beat Candida Cookbook

Water to cover

2 tbsp fine oatmeal mixed with 8 tbsp cold water

4 tbsp tomato purée (no citric acid)

1 tsp dried mixed herbs

2 cans of kidney or haricot beans, or chickpeas (garbanzos) (no sugar)

Lightly cook the vegetables in water which just covers them. When tender, mix the oatmeal and water in a bowl, then add some of the hot vegetable juice to it, stirring carefully. When the paste is smooth, add it to the hot water with the vegetables, stirring all the time. Cook for two minutes, till the gravy is thick, then stir in the tomato purée and herbs. Lastly, drain and thoroughly rinse the beans, then tip them in with the vegetables and heat through gently, making sure that the gravy doesn't 'catch' on the bottom.

✳✳✳ Bean and Vegetable Pie

Prepare a pot of stew as above, and stop cooking while the vegetables are still fairly firm because they will get more cooking in the pie. Make one batch of Shortcrust Wholemeal Pastry *(see page 99)*, and line a round quiche dish with it. Fill with the stew and add a pastry lid, sealing the edges and cutting slits to allow the steam to escape. Bake at 375°F/190°C/Gas Mark 5 for 30–40 minutes.

✳✳✳ Bean and Vegetable Cobbler

Make a potful of Bean and Vegetable Stew as in one of the previous recipes, put it into a casserole or pie dish, then make little scones to put on the top as follows:

225g/8oz/1½ cups wholemeal flour

1 tsp potassium (or sodium) bicarbonate

3 tbsp extra virgin olive oil (or unrefined sunflower oil)

300ml/½ pint/1⅓ cups soya milk (or rice milk)

2 tbsp fresh lemon juice

Poppy seeds

Preheat oven to 375°F/190°C/Gas Mark 5. Sift together flour and bicarbonate powder, then mix in the oil. Stir in the soya milk and lemon juice and mix to a soft dough with a fork. Roll out on a well-floured surface and cut into 6cm/2½-inch rounds with a pastry cutter or top of a glass. Brush the tops with soya milk and sprinkle with poppy seeds. Arrange on top of the vegetables and bake for 30 minutes, or microwave on High for 10 minutes.

*** Bean and Vegetable Stew with Dumplings

Make a potful of Bean and Vegetable Stew as in one of the previous recipes and use the recipe for dumplings which follows.

*** Lemony Chickpeas (Garbanzos) with Dumplings

125g/4oz/1 cup green pepper, deseeded and sliced
1 medium onion, chopped
125g/4 oz/1 cup aubergine (eggplant), chopped
1 tbsp extra virgin olive oil
1 lemon, squeezed
2 tbsp chopped parsley
225g/8oz/1 cup chickpeas (garbanzos), soaked and cooked (or 1–2 cans cooked chickpeas)
450ml/¾ pint/2 cups vegetable stock (or 2 tsp tomato purée in 450ml/¾ pint/2 cups boiling water)
Freshly ground black pepper

Dumplings:
125g/4oz/1 scant cup wholemeal flour
½ tsp potassium (or sodium) bicarbonate
1 tbsp extra virgin olive oil (or unrefined sunflower oil)
1 tsp fresh lemon juice
Cold filtered water
1 tbsp sesame seeds

Preheat oven to 375°F/190°C/Gas Mark 5. Soften green pepper, onion and aubergine in the oil for a few minutes over a low heat, then stir in the lemon juice and parsley. Cover and cook over low heat for 3 minutes then put into a large casserole dish with the cooked chickpeas (garbanzos). Heat the stock to boiling point in a saucepan (or add boiling water to tomato purée), season with freshly ground black pepper, and pour over chickpeas (garbanzos) and vegetables.

To make dumplings, sift the flour and bicarbonate together, mix in the oil and lemon juice and stir in enough cold water to make a firm dough. With your hands, make 8 little balls. Put some sesame seeds into a saucer and roll the dumplings in them, pressing slightly to make sure they stick. Put the dumplings in the casserole on top of the chickpeas (garbanzos) and vegetables. Bake for 30 minutes, or cook in the microwave on High for 5 minutes.

*** Bean Paella

GLUTEN-FREE

250g/8oz/1½ cups (dried weight) red kidney beans (or 2 cans beans, sugar-free)
250g/8oz/1¼ cups long-grain whole rice
450ml/¾ pint/2 cups water
½ tsp turmeric
2 tbsp extra virgin olive oil
1 large onion, chopped
1 green pepper, deseeded and chopped
2 sticks celery, chopped
2 large carrots, chopped
1 small aubergine (eggplant), chopped
1 clove garlic, crushed
4 large tomatoes, peeled and chopped (or 1 medium can tomatoes)
2 tbsp chopped fresh parsley
Freshly ground black pepper

Soak and cook the beans as described on pages 167–9. Wash the rice and put in a large pan with the water and turmeric. Bring to the boil, cover and simmer gently on a low heat for 30 minutes. Meanwhile, put the oil in another pan with the onion, pepper, celery, carrots, aubergine (eggplant) and garlic and cook over a low heat for 10 minutes, stirring frequently, then add the tomatoes. Heat through for 5 minutes, then tip the vegetables in with the rice, add the cooked beans, cover and leave over a very low heat for another 10 minutes. Stir with a fork, and add the ground pepper and parsley before serving.

*** Bean and Courgette (Zucchini) Pie

1 batch of wholemeal pastry (see page 99)
2 medium onions, sliced
1 clove garlic, crushed
675g/1½lb/6 cups courgettes (zucchini), sliced
1 tbsp extra virgin olive oil
6 tomatoes, skinned and chopped, or 1 medium can tomatoes
1 tbsp tomato purée (no citric acid)
Herbs or spices to taste
225g/8oz (dried weight) any type beans, soaked and cooked (or 1–2 cans cooked beans,
    sugar-free, rinsed)

Preheat oven to 400°F/200°C/Gas Mark 6. Prepare the pastry. Cook onions, garlic and courgettes (zucchini) in the oil over a low heat for 10 minutes. Add tomatoes, tomato purée and seasonings, cover and simmer for 5 minutes. Add the cooked beans and stir. Line a flan tin with pastry, add the bean and vegetable mixture, roll out more pastry and make a lid for the pie. Press well together round the edges, cut a few slits in the top to allow steam to escape, decorate with pastry leaves and bake for 25–30 minutes.

* Slow-Cooker Spicy Beans

GLUTEN-FREE

2 medium onions, chopped
1 or 2 medium cans red kidney beans (sugar-free, rinsed)
2 courgettes (zucchini), washed and sliced
1 medium can tomatoes (no citric acid)
1 tsp ground cumin
1 tsp ground coriander

Preheat the slow-cooker on High. Heat all ingredients in a saucepan then turn into the slow-cooker. Turn cooker to Low and leave all day. Serve with whole-grain rice.

* Quick Home-made 'Baked Beans'

GLUTEN-FREE

2 onions
1 tbsp extra virgin olive oil
400g/14oz can tomatoes (no citric acid)
2 tbsp tomato purée (no citric acid)
1 tsp mixed herbs and 1 tsp paprika
Freshly ground black pepper
1 medium can haricot beans in salt water (sugar-free)

Finely chop onions and soften in oil over gentle heat. Add tomatoes, tomato purée, herbs, paprika and pepper. Stir well, mashing tomatoes, and simmer for a few minutes to obtain a fairly thick sauce. If you want it to be smooth, put it through a blender. Drain and rinse the beans and add to the sauce. Heat through, and serve in a baked potato or on toasted gluten-free potato bread (*page 267*) or soda bread (*pages 73–4*). Can also be eaten cold with salad.

** (*) Provençal Beans

GLUTEN-FREE

350g/12oz/1¾ cups haricot or other beans, soaked and cooked (or 1–2 cans cooked beans, sugar-free)
2 medium onions, sliced
1 red pepper, deseeded and sliced
1 green pepper, deseeded and sliced
1 or 2 cloves garlic, crushed
2 tbsp extra virgin olive oil
400g/14oz can tomatoes (no citric acid)
2 tbsp tomato purée (no citric acid)
Large pinch of mixed herbs
300ml/½ pint/1⅓ cups boiling water

Freshly ground black pepper
2 tbsp chopped fresh parsley

Soak and cook the beans (*see pages 166–9*), or empty the canned beans into a colander and rinse thoroughly. Soften onions, peppers and garlic in the oil over a low heat for 10 minutes, add the contents of the tin of tomatoes, tomato purée, herbs, beans and water. Season with pepper, cover and simmer till heated right through, 20–30 minutes. Add parsley just before the end.

** Bean Burgers

MAY BE GLUTEN-FREE

1 medium onion, finely chopped
2 tomatoes, skinned and chopped
1 large can beans, drained and rinsed
1 medium carrot, grated
125g/4oz/1 cup ground seeds (sunflower, pumpkin or sesame)
50g/2oz/1¾ cups porridge oats
2 tbsp tomato purée
4 tbsp chopped fresh parsley (or ½ tsp any dried herbs)
1 tsp yeast-free vegetable bouillon
Wholemeal flour to coat
Optional for gluten-free version: coat with buckwheat flour or rice flour instead of whole-
    meal flour

Preheat oven to 400°F/200°C/Gas Mark 6. Soften onion in covered pan over low heat or else in microwave, adding tomatoes at the end. Mash the beans and mix all ingredients together. Form into 8 burgers, coat with flour and place on floured baking tray. Bake for 20 minutes.

Erica White's Beat Candida Cookbook

** Bean Bake

GLUTEN-FREE

1 onion, diced
1 clove garlic, chopped.
1 tbsp extra virgin olive oil
3 beef tomatoes, skinned and chopped
350g/12oz/2 cups any cooked beans e.g. red kidney, chickpeas (garbanzos), black-eyed
    beans (or 1 can of any beans, sugar-free, rinsed)
1 tsp mixed dried herbs
Freshly ground black pepper

Preheat oven to 350°F/180°C/Gas Mark 4. Sauté onion and garlic in oil. Add chopped tomatoes, beans, herbs and black pepper. Put in a covered dish and bake for 35 minutes. Serve with brown rice and a green vegetable.

** Kidney Bean and Potato Pie

GLUTEN-FREE

2 large onions, peeled and diced
1 tbsp extra virgin olive oil
425g/15oz/2½ cups tomatoes, skinned and chopped (or 1 medium can tomatoes, no citric
    acid)
225g/8oz/1⅓ cups red kidney beans, soaked and cooked (or 1 medium can beans, sugar-
    free, rinsed)
Freshly ground black pepper
25g/1oz/knob unsalted butter
2 tbsp soya milk (or rice milk)
¾kg/1½lb/4½ cups cooked, mashed potatoes

Preheat oven to 400°F/200°C/Gas Mark 6. Sauté onions in oil until soft. Remove from heat and add tomatoes, beans and pepper. Put into casserole dish. Mix butter and soya milk into mashed potato and put on top of bean mixture. Bake for 40 minutes or until golden brown. Serve grated cheese separately for non-candida dieters.

---

* Falafel

GLUTEN-FREE

225g/8oz/1 cup chickpeas (garbanzos), soaked and cooked (or 1 medium can, sugar-free, rinsed)
1 free-range egg
1 onion, finely chopped
2 tbsp fresh parsley, chopped
1 clove garlic, crushed
1 tsp ground coriander
1 tsp ground cumin
Freshly ground black pepper
Buckwheat flour for moulding
2 tbsp extra virgin olive oil

Put all ingredients except buckwheat flour and oil into food processor and blend until mostly smooth. Mix with buckwheat flour to a consistency that will shape into patties. Shallow fry in the oil for 3 minutes on each side. Stand on kitchen paper on a plate in a low oven to keep warm. Serve with brown rice and salad.

---

* Lentil Wedges

GLUTEN-FREE

225g/8oz/1 cup red lentils
450ml/¾ pint/2 cups water
1 large onion, diced
1 tbsp extra virgin olive oil
1 tsp dried mixed herbs
1 free-range egg
Freshly ground black pepper

Preheat oven to 375°F/190°C/Gas Mark 5. Cook the lentils in the water until soft and no liquid is left. Sauté onion in oil until soft. Combine all ingredients and press into a 22cm/9-inch sandwich tin lined with greaseproof paper. Bake for 30 minutes. Serve hot or cold.

** Lentil Burgers

225g/8oz/1 cup red lentils
600ml/1 pint/2½ cups water
2 large carrots, grated
1 large onion, chopped
4 tbsp wholemeal flour
1 tsp mixed herbs
Freshly grated nutmeg
Freshly ground black pepper

Rinse and sort lentils, then place in a small saucepan, cover with water and bring to the boil. Put lid on pan, reduce heat and simmer gently till lentils are cooked and water absorbed (15–20 minutes). Leave to cool. Preheat oven to 400°F/200°C/Gas Mark 6. Put lentils into a bowl, add carrots, onion, flour, herbs, nutmeg and pepper. Mix well. Shape into 8 burgers, put on floured baking tray and bake for 15–20 minutes.

* Lentil Bolognese Sauce

GLUTEN-FREE IF NOT ADDED TO PASTA

1 medium onion, sliced
1 stick celery, chopped
½ green pepper, deseeded and chopped
1 tbsp extra virgin olive oil
175g/6oz/1 scant cup brown lentils
425g/15oz can tomatoes (no citric acid)
2 bay leaves
1 tsp cinnamon

I tsp mixed herbs
Water to cover

In a large saucepan, soften the onion, celery and pepper in the oil over a low heat for 1 minute. Rinse the lentils and pick over for stones. Add lentils, tomatoes and other ingredients to the saucepan and add sufficient water to cover. Bring to the boil, then put lid on pan and simmer over a low heat for 20–30 minutes, adding more water if necessary. Serve with wholewheat pasta shells or spaghetti, cooked in boiling water for 12 minutes.

** Lentil Lasagne

The recipe for Lentil Bolognese can be used with pre-cooked sheets of wholewheat lasagne. Prepare the sauce and preheat the oven to 375°F/190°C/Gas Mark 5. Put 3 or 4 tablespoons of lentil sauce into the bottom of a casserole dish, then arrange a layer of pasta sheets, add more lentil sauce, and so on, ending with lasagne. On top of this put yoghurt sauce, made as follows, and bake in the oven for 40 minutes.

---

* Yoghurt Sauce for Lasagne Topping

2 free-range eggs
300ml/½ pint/1⅓ cups natural yoghurt
Freshly ground black pepper
Optional: 25g/1oz/1 tbsp wholemeal flour (for a thicker sauce)
Optional: 1 small packet of plain crisps

Beat the eggs, mix in the yoghurt and pepper (and flour if used). Pour on top of the lentil lasagne. If liked, crush a bag of plain crisps and sprinkle on top. Bake as directed for Lentil Lasagne.

Seeds

The most usual seeds to use for baking purposes are the larger varieties, sunflower and pumpkin, but sesame seeds can also be used. They are high in protein, vitamins, minerals and essential fatty acids. You do need a grinder, though.

---

* Seed Rissoles

GLUTEN-FREE, MAKES 4

50g/2oz/⅓ cup pumpkin seeds
50g/2oz/⅓ cup sunflower seeds
50g/2oz/⅓ cup sesame seeds
2 sticks celery, chopped
¼ tsp ground cumin
¼ tsp turmeric
½ lemon, squeezed
1 tbsp chopped parsley

Grind the seeds thoroughly, and mix in with all the other ingredients. Blend in a food processor until the mixture binds. Shape into rissoles and they're ready to serve with salad; no cooking required!

** Seed Loaf

1 cup bulgar
1 cup water
¾ cup sunflower seeds
1 medium onion
2 tomatoes
2 tbsp soya flour
1 tbsp rice flour
Herbs

Freshly ground black pepper
Juice from can of tomatoes (no citric acid) or water to mix

Using extra virgin olive oil or unsalted butter, oil a loaf tin, line with greaseproof paper and oil again. Preheat oven to 375°F/190°C/Gas Mark 5. To cook bulgar, add 1 cup of water, bring to boil and leave to stand for 15 minutes. Grind the sunflower seeds. Gently soften the onion and one of the tomatoes in a covered pan or microwave. Mix all ingredients together, adding enough tomato juice or water to obtain a sticky mixture. Slice the remaining tomato and make a row along the bottom of the loaf tin. Put the mixture on top, pressing down firmly. Bake for 40 minutes or until firm. Turn out of tin and remove paper, so that the row of tomatoes is on top. Serve hot or cold.

This recipe could equally well use nuts as seeds, but nuts do tend to have invisible mould on them once they have been shelled, so it's not a good idea to buy them in packets from the health-food store, and not many people will want to sit and crack a pile of nuts before they grind them for a recipe. However, you can if you like!

Chapter 24

Meat and Poultry

There really is no need to include basic recipes for meat and poultry in an anti-candida cookbook because they present no problems – except that you need to remember not to put mushrooms in a casserole, not to use hot spices like chilli or curry, not to make exotic sauces containing wine, cider, vinegar or cream, not to put cheese on top of pasta and not to use a gravy mix containing yeast or monosodium glutamate.

The other point to remember is that most meat will have residues of antibiotics and hormones in it unless the animal has been reared by organic farming methods. The least likely to be affected is lamb, but even so it is good to track down a butcher who sells organically reared meat if possible, because this will ensure that it is free of hormone and antibiotic residues, and also that it has not been treated with artificial preservatives and colourings. The bright red colour of the meat in many shop windows is simply too dazzling to be true!

Free-range chickens are getting much easier to obtain, and even the large supermarkets have realized the demand for them and usually stock a few frozen ones. However, nothing can beat the taste and texture of a fresh free-range chicken, so do ask around at your local butchers' shops.

The cost of organic meat and free-range chicken is certainly more than you would otherwise pay, but if you are embarking on new eating habits which include fish of various sorts and dishes made with dried beans and lentils, you will find that the lower costs of meals overall will allow your budget to stretch to really good meat on the few days that you eat it.

Since cold cooked meats without preservatives are difficult to find, and ham is excluded in the diet, it can be helpful to have some cold meat in the refrigerator the day after you've cooked it, but there are a few other factors to be borne in mind when you consider eating red meats.

All red meat, however lean, contains a high percentage of animal fat. This saturated fat is not only a disadvantage from the point of view of calories and cholesterol, but it also contains arachidonic acid, which is an inflammatory substance. If you are trying to reduce aches and pains of any description you would do well to avoid red meat as much as possible. It also causes an imbalance of essential fatty acids, because most people have too little of the right sort of oils in their diet, and this can lead to problems with hormonal situations (PMT and period irregularities in particular), skin conditions like eczema, clogging of the arteries and lowered immunity.

The general rule to follow about red meat is that if you really like it and are not suffering with any of the health problems mentioned above, eat it no more than twice a week and try to make sure that you are buying it from an 'organic' butcher. Otherwise avoid it. Chicken is white meat but the skin is very high in saturated fat and gives the same problems as red meat. If you can find free-range chicken, you might like to include it in your menus twice a week, avoiding the skin.

Although I have said that you don't need special recipes for cooking meat and poultry, nevertheless I sometimes find that clients leave my consulting room after their first visit feeling there is absolutely *nothing* they can eat on the anti-candida diet, and I need to point out to them that with main meals there is actually very little problem. So to encourage you to discover this for yourself, I include a few recipes for lamb and chicken.

Straightforward roasting in the oven is obviously extremely easy, and it does have the advantage of giving you some cold meat to cut, but don't leave it in the refrigerator for longer than a day because it will start to gather unseen mould. It's a good idea to slice your meat or chicken when it is cold, and then freeze the ready-cooked, ready-sliced cold meat in handy-sized portions. Make sure it is completely thawed before you eat it, and don't be tempted to thaw it in the microwave. Meat or poultry which becomes just warm, rather than really heated through, creates just the conditions which bugs enjoy – and food poisoning is *all* you need!

---

* Roast Lamb

Preheat oven to 400°F/200°C/Gas Mark 6. Weigh the meat and work out the cooking time as follows: 20 minutes per ½ kg/1lb plus 20 minutes extra. Put a little water in the bottom of the pan; it doesn't need extra fat. Cook in the centre of the oven for the required time. You can poke a few leaves of fresh herbs into the meat before cooking to give it a lovely aromatic flavour; try rosemary, thyme or sage. Test the meat with a knife or skewer to make sure that the juices are no longer red, then allow to stand for a few minutes before carving.

Roast Free-range Poultry

Not many people now have to pluck, draw and truss their poultry before they can cook and eat it, so be thankful! However, there are some precautions you need to take if, once again, you want to avoid the risk of food poisoning.

If using frozen poultry, it must be thoroughly thawed in the refrigerator (at least 28 hours for a 900g/2lb bird or 44 hours for 2.25kg/5lb) or at room temperature (at least 8 hours for a small bird or 12–16 hours for 2.25kg/5lb–3.15kg/7lb – or even longer, depending on the size of the bird). For large turkeys, see page 186.

If buying a fresh turkey from the butcher, always ask for the giblets. These will give you delicious stock or gravy, and are good to eat as well. For some reason, chicken giblets are no longer allowed to be sold, which is a great pity. Wash and weigh the prepared bird; if you are going to stuff it using one of the recipes in Chapter 19 'Sauces and Stuffings', the total weight of the stuffed bird should be allowed in the cooking time. Put a little water in the bottom of the pan; no fat is necessary, but you might like to put a piece of butter paper over the breast to stop it being overcooked on top. Cooking times are given below. When testing, the juices should run clear and watery – not red.

---

* Roast Chicken

Preheat oven to 400°F/200°C/Gas Mark 6. Prepare as above. Cook for 20 minutes per ½kg/1lb, including weight of stuffing.

---

* Roast Duck or Goose

Preheat oven to 400°F/200°C/Gas Mark 6. Prepare as above. These birds are fatty, so prick the skin well all over to allow the fat to run out, and cook on a grid in the roasting pan, so that the bird is not standing in the fat. A goose can produce so much fat that you may need to pour it out of the tin at intervals during the cooking time. Cook for 20 minutes per ½ kg/1lb, including weight of stuffing.

---

* Roast Turkey

Preheat oven to 325°F/170°C/Gas Mark 3 for frozen turkeys, or for fresh turkeys, preheat oven to 425°F/220°C/Gas Mark 7. Frozen turkeys may take 36–66 hours to thaw at room temperature, depending on size. Prepare as above. Put a little water in the bottom of the pan, spread butter all over the bird and cover with some greaseproof paper. Calculate the cooking time as follows, and include the weight of the stuffing in the time needed:

Defrosted frozen turkey, weight including stuffing, at 325°F/160°C/Gas Mark 3

2¾–4½ kg/6–10lb	3–3¾ hours
4½–6¼ kg/10–14lb	3¾–4¼ hours
6¼–8¼ kg/14–18lb	4¼–4¾ hours
8¼–10kg/18–22lb	4¾–5 hours

Fresh turkey, weight including stuffing, at 425°F/220°C/Gas Mark 7

2¾–4½ kg/6–10lb	2½–2¾ hours
4½–6¼ kg/10–14lb	2¾–3¼ hours
6¼–8¼ kg/14–18lb	3¼–3¾ hours
8¼–10kg/18–22lb	3¾–4 hours

---

* Turkey Giblet Stock or Gravy

GLUTEN-FREE

Wash and trim the giblets, taking off any surplus fat, peeling the hard skin from the gizzard and trimming off any yellow patches from the liver, which make it bitter. Slice an onion, a carrot and a stick of celery. Put everything in a saucepan and cover with cold water. Add freshly ground black pepper and a pinch of herbs. Bring to the boil quickly, then reduce the heat, cover the pan and simmer gently for 30–40 minutes.

Chicken Dishes

Free-range chicken provides good protein value in the form of white meat, which does not have the inflammatory properties of red meat provided you remove the skin in order to reduce its fat content. As many chicken meals take very little time and energy to prepare, it is worth having a wide variety of recipes so that you can ring the changes.

* Simple Chicken Casserole

GLUTEN-FREE

Preheat oven to 350°F/180°C/Gas Mark 4. Wash chicken and put it whole into a large casserole dish. Around it put a sliced onion, sliced carrots, pieces of potato, sliced green pepper or other vegetables – as many as you like or there is room for! Add mixed herbs and freshly ground black pepper, then pour on plenty of boiling water, enough to cover the vegetables, and put the lid on the casserole dish. Cook in the oven for 1½–2 hours. This makes an extremely easy and tasty all-in-one meal, and will provide extra meat for the next day as well as a jug of stock or soup. If you have many vegetables left over, liquidize them and add to the stock to make a good thick broth.

* Chicken Portions with Tarragon

GLUTEN-FREE

This recipe can be made with very little energy using frozen vegetables, and may either be casseroled in the oven as the previous recipe or left all day in a slow-cooker.

2 medium onions, chopped
I clove garlic, crushed (or ½ tsp garlic granules)
I mug frozen sweetcorn
I mug frozen carrot slices
I medium can tomatoes (no citric acid)
4 chicken joints, skinned
2 tbsp chopped fresh tarragon
Freshly ground black pepper

Preheat the slow-cooker on High. Heat all ingredients in a saucepan, transfer to slow-cooker and switch to Low. Leave all day. Alternatively, preheat the oven to 350°F/180°C/ Gas Mark 4, put all ingredients into a casserole dish, cover and cook for 2–3 hours. This way, you can put in some scrubbed potatoes to bake at the same time; be sure to prick them first.

Lemon Chicken

I received many recipes for lemon-flavoured chicken, but the following four recipes show different ways of cooking it.

---

* Lemon Bay Chicken

GLUTEN-FREE

I x 1.5kg/3½ lb chicken
½ tsp paprika
½ tsp garlic granules
½ tsp ground bay leaves
½ organic lemon
I carton Greek or strained yoghurt

Preheat the oven to 375°C/190°C/Gas Mark 5. Wash and trim the chicken, removing any surplus fat, and place in a roasting dish. Sprinkle with the herbs and spices, squeeze the juice from the lemon all over it and put the lemon 'shell' in the body cavity (this adds flavour and moisture, but make sure the lemon is well scrubbed). Cover the chicken with some buttered greaseproof paper, and cook for 1½ hours. When ready, lift the chicken onto a warmed plate, strain the fat off the juices and add the yoghurt to them. Carve the chicken and serve it with the yoghurt sauce.

---

* Baked Lemon Chicken Breasts

GLUTEN-FREE

2 organic lemons
4 chicken breasts, skinned

Scrub the lemons and grate the rinds, then squeeze out their juice. Marinate the chicken breasts with the lemon juice and grated rind in a covered bowl overnight in the refrigerator. Preheat oven to 375°F/190°C/Gas Mark 5. Place chicken breasts on an oiled baking sheet and bake for ¾–1 hour, or until thoroughly cooked and golden. You could bake jacket potatoes at the same time and serve them with cottage cheese and have a crisp green salad as a side dish.

** Lemon Chicken

GLUTEN-FREE

1 clove garlic
1 organic lemon
450g/1lb/2 cups chicken breasts, cubed
1 tbsp extra virgin olive oil
175ml/6fl oz/¾ cup filtered water
1 tbsp maize flour

Crush the garlic and scrub and grate the lemon, then squeeze out its juice. Cook chicken in oil in a deep pan for 2 minutes, stirring. Add garlic, lemon rind and lemon juice. Mix maize flour with some of the water, gradually mixing in and adding all the water, and then bring to the boil in a small pan, stirring until thickened. Add to chicken and simmer on a low heat for about 25 minutes until cooked. Serve with brown rice and a green vegetable.

---

* Lemon Turkey Steaks or Chicken Joints

GLUTEN-FREE

Turkey steaks or chicken joints, quantity as required
Juice of 1 lemon
Rosemary or thyme, fresh or dried.

Preheat oven to 325°F/170°C/Gas Mark 3. Put meat in a casserole dish, pour the lemon juice over it and sprinkle with herbs. Put on the lid and cook for 1½ hours or until tender.

** Chicken or Lamb Kebabs

GLUTEN-FREE

600ml/1 pint/2½ cups natural yoghurt
1 clove garlic, crushed (or ½ tsp garlic granules)
Juice of 1 lemon
Freshly ground black pepper
450g/1 lb/2 cups chicken or lamb cut into cubes
2 medium onions
1 green pepper
1 red or yellow pepper
225g/½ lb cherry tomatoes
4 metal kebab skewers

Make a marinade from the yoghurt, garlic, lemon and seasoning. Soak the meat cubes in it for 2–3 hours. Prepare the vegetables by slicing the onion downwards and cutting the washed peppers into 8 sections each, removing all seeds. Wash the cherry tomatoes. Thread everything onto the skewers, alternating cubes of meat with pieces of onion, pepper and tomatoes, ending with a tomato. Brush all over with the marinade, and cook under a hot grill for 15–20 minutes, turning several times. Serve with brown rice.

Erica White's Beat Candida Cookbook

** Chicken Risotto

GLUTEN-FREE

2 tbsp extra virgin olive oil
225g/8oz/1 cup brown rice
450g/1lb/2 cups chicken breasts, cubed
125g/4oz/1 scant cup carrot, diced
1 large onion, finely chopped
1 tsp paprika
1 tbsp tomato purée (no citric acid)
2 beef tomatoes, skinned and chopped
125ml/4fl oz/½ cup water

Heat the oil in a deep pan and add half the rice, cooking for 3 minutes on low heat. Add the carrot and onion and cook for 3 more minutes. Add the chicken and cook for 3 further minutes, stirring. Add everything else and stir. Simmer for 45 minutes or until the rice is cooked and all the liquid has been absorbed. Cook the remaining rice separately to serve with the risotto and a green vegetable.

* Chicken and Tarragon Burgers

MAY BE WHEAT-FREE, MAKES 6

450g/1 lb/2 cups minced raw chicken
1 onion
Fresh tarragon, roughly chopped – as much as liked
85g/3oz/1 cup rolled oats
Flour for dusting – any type – wheat, rye, potato, gram or rice

Mix the chicken, onion, tarragon and oats together until mixture does not cling to sides of the bowl. The mixture is moist so nothing should be needed to bind it. Dust surface with flour and shape tablespoonsful of mixture into small round cakes about 8cm/3 inches in diameter and 2cm/¾-inch thick. Place on a greased baking tray and cook at 375°F/190°C/Gas Mark 5, turning regularly, for about 45 minutes or until insides look cooked. Can be served with jacket potatoes and stir-fried vegetables, or cold with a salad, or in a soda bread roll with home-made tomato sauce if you are pining for a burger!

Using Cooked Chicken

Cooked chicken can be used in many ways, such as in a variety of quiche fillings. Since the basic ingredient of a quiche is usually eggs or tofu, recipes can be found in Chapter 26, starting on page 208, and some basic ideas you will find there for quiche fillings are Chicken and Cucumber, Chicken and Avocado and Chicken and Broccoli.

---

* Quick Chicken or Turkey Pilaff

GLUTEN-FREE

Here is another way of using leftover cooked chicken or turkey.

3–4 chicken joints, cooked, or leftovers from cooked chicken OR
cooked turkey, quantity as required per person
1 tbsp extra virgin olive oil (or 25g/1oz/knob unsalted butter)
1 medium onion, peeled and chopped
225g/8oz/1 cup wholegrain rice
600ml/1 pint/2½ cups hot stock (chicken, turkey or vegetable)
1 bay leaf

Remove meat from joints or carcass and chop into bite sizes. Put the oil or butter into a saucepan with the onion and cook gently over a low heat for a few minutes, till the onion is soft. Stir in the rice and stock, add the bay leaf and bring to the boil. Cover, reduce heat and simmer gently for 30 minutes or until the rice is tender and the liquid has been absorbed. Add the pieces of meat, heat through thoroughly for about 5 minutes, stirring to prevent 'catching'.

Lamb Dishes

Just to show you that I am not totally averse to red meat (provided your body can cope with eating it), here are a couple more recipes for lamb. Any of these dishes could be made with brown lentils instead, and I know which I prefer, both for flavour and for health!

*** Moussaka

3 medium-sized aubergines (eggplants)
Extra virgin olive oil
1 large onion, sliced
450g/1lb/2 cups minced lamb
150ml/¼ pint/⅔ cup vegetable stock or 1 small can tomatoes (no citric acid)
Freshly ground black pepper

Sauce for Topping:
2 free-range eggs
300ml/½ pint/1⅓ cups natural yoghurt
25g/1oz wholemeal flour

Wash the aubergines (eggplants) and cut into 6cm/¼-inch thick slices. Brush with a little oil, place on a lightly oiled baking tray and put under the grill for 5 minutes, turning when golden brown. Soften the onion in a large pan over a low heat, using the minimum of oil if needed. Add the lamb and cook until browned, 15–20 minutes. Stir in the stock or tin of tomatoes and black pepper, and simmer gently for 15–20 minutes. Now preheat the oven to 350°F/180°C/Gas Mark 4. When all ingredients are ready, put a layer of aubergines (eggplants) into a casserole dish and add half the lamb mixture. Add another layer of aubergines (eggplants), then the rest of the lamb, and finish with a layer of aubergines (eggplants). Make the sauce by beating the eggs and adding the yoghurt and wholemeal flour. Pour the sauce over the aubergines (eggplants) and bake for 30 minutes. For family or visitors who are not on the anti-candida diet, you can grate some cheese to add when serving, and this will melt into the sauce.

*** Lamb Layer Pie

This is very similar to Moussaka but has a less 'exotic' taste, using sliced cooked potatoes and sliced tomatoes instead of aubergines (eggplants) to make the layers. Allow 450g/1lb/3¼ cups potatoes and 225g/½lb/1⅓ cups tomatoes to every 225g/½lb/1 cup of minced lamb. Cook in the same way as Moussaka.

** Lamb Lasagne

Another variation on the theme can be made using the same ingredients as Moussaka but using precooked wholewheat lasagne sheets instead of aubergine (eggplants). Also, add some mixed herbs or oregano to the lamb mixture. Layer in the same way, ending with sauce, which can exclude the flour if you like a thinner topping. Cook in the same way, allowing 35–40 minutes.

* Lamb Burgers

GLUTEN-FREE

450g/1lb/2 cups minced lamb
1 free-range egg, beaten
2 tbsp fresh mint, chopped
2 tbsp fresh parsley, chopped
Freshly ground black pepper

Mix all ingredients together, divide into 8 and make into burger shapes. Cook under medium grill for about 7 minutes each side. (Freeze uncooked with greaseproof paper layers.)

** Cornish Pasties

For 4 pasties allow:

2 small onions, finely chopped
2 small carrots, finely chopped
2 small potatoes, finely chopped
2 tsp extra virgin olive oil
125g/4oz/½ cup minced lamb
Freshly ground black pepper
1 batch Wholemeal Shortcrust Pastry (page 99) or Oaty Pastry (page 100)
Optional: egg to glaze

Gently 'sweat' the chopped onions, carrots and potatoes in the oil over a low heat for 5 minutes, until softened. Add lamb and black pepper and cook till brown, 10–15 minutes. Preheat oven to 400°F/200°C/Gas Mark 6. Make the pastry, divide into four and roll each into an 18cm/7-inch round. Arrange the filling down the centre of each round, dampen the pastry edges and bring them to meet above the filling, pressing together and fluting with finger and thumb. Place on an oiled baking tray, glaze with egg if using and bake for 20 minutes. Serve hot or cold.

*** Greek Pastitsio

SERVES 4–6

What better way to end the meat recipes than with spicy lamb, the way the Greeks eat it? This is sure to impress your friends!

450g/1lb/2 cups lean minced lamb
1 large onion, finely chopped
1 clove garlic, crushed
1 tsp dried oregano
½ tsp ground cinnamon
1 tsp ground cumin
Pinch of ground ginger
Pinch of grated nutmeg
1 bay leaf
150ml/¼ pint/⅔ cup vegetable stock
400g/14oz can chopped tomatoes (no citric acid)
1 tbsp tomato purée (no citric acid)
Freshly ground black pepper
175g/6oz/2 cups wholewheat pasta
Optional: 2 tbsp freshly chopped coriander
25g/1oz unsalted butter (or 1 tbsp extra virgin olive oil)
25g/1oz soya flour
350ml/12fl oz/1½ cups soya milk
1 free-range egg, beaten

Place mince in a large non-stick pan with the onion and garlic, and cook over a moderate heat for 5 minutes until browned. Stir in the herbs, spices and bay leaf and cook for a further 5 minutes, stirring occasionally. Stir in the vegetable stock, tomatoes, tomato purée and seasoning. Bring to the boil, half cover and simmer for 30 minutes, stirring occasionally until the sauce is thickened and well reduced. Meanwhile, preheat the oven to 375°/190°/Gas Mark 5 and also cook the pasta in boiling water until just tender. Drain and stir into the lamb mixture with the chopped coriander, if using. Now spoon into a large shallow 1 litre/2-pint ovenproof dish.

Place the butter or oil with the soya flour and soya milk in a saucepan and whisk continuously over a moderate heat until thickened. Remove from the heat and allow to cool slightly. Beat in the egg and season to taste with freshly ground black pepper. Pour this sauce over the lamb mixture and cook in the oven for 35–40 minutes. Serve hot with a green salad and crusty soda bread.

Chapter 25

Fish

As with meat and poultry, there really is no need for a section on fish in an anti-candida recipe book, because it presents no problem to the yeasty person, unless it is smoked. However, I'm including a few ideas just to whet your appetite.

Actually, I feel sad about fish because it ought to be one of the most nourishing and health-building foods available to us, instead of which it is full of pollutants which we take in every time we eat it. The sea around Britain is full of industrial waste and chemical toxins, but personally, I would rather take good levels of vitamins and minerals each day to detoxify the major effects of this type of pollution than have to avoid fish for the rest of my life.

It is said that frozen fish is probably less polluted than fresh fish because it has been caught in areas of the world which are less heavily populated. This is worth thinking about, and certainly frozen fish is extremely useful to keep in the freezer, but I still feel there is nothing quite like the flavour and texture of a fresh herring or mackerel, or a plaice straight from the sea.

There are two main types of fish available to us: white fish like cod, haddock, huss and plaice; and oily fish like herring, sardines, mackerel and salmon. Canned fish like pilchards and tuna are also oily fish, and although we should try to keep canned food to a minimum, fish is one of the best excuses for buying it. Deciding whether to buy it in oil or in brine is a question of choosing the lesser evil, but I prefer brine because the oils used are cheap, refined oils which can do a lot of damage. Oily fish is an extremely beneficial food. Not only does it counteract the inflammatory fats found in meat and dairy produce but it can also help to reduce blood pressure by keeping the arteries clear and preventing blood from becoming too sticky. Studies have shown that people with high blood pressure or a history of stroke or heart problems do very well when they include plenty of oily fish in their diet.

Tuna

Canned tuna is a useful ingredient for some main meal recipes, as well as being good eaten cold with a salad. Several clients have sent me recipes for varieties of tuna quiche, and some of these will be found in Chapter 26. Tuna quiches can be served either cold or hot.

---

* Tuna Bake

This useful hot dish is very easy to prepare.

200g/7oz can tuna in brine, drained well
225g/8oz/1 cup cottage cheese
225g/8oz/2 cups courgettes (zucchini), washed and sliced
150g/5oz/1¾ cups wholemeal pasta (any type), cooked
350g/12oz/2 cups skinned tomatoes, puréed (or 1 medium can tomatoes without the juice)
Fresh chopped herbs to taste (try basil or dill)

Preheat oven to 375°F/190°C/Gas Mark 5. Mix tuna with cottage cheese. Grease a casserole dish and put in courgettes (zucchini), pasta, and the tuna/cottage cheese mixture. Pour the puréed tomatoes over and sprinkle with fresh herbs. Bake for 30–35 minutes, till courgettes (zucchini) are tender.

---

* Tuna and Tomato Topping

GLUTEN-FREE
This is quick and useful for serving on a baked potato or some wholemeal pasta – or on toasted wholemeal soda bread.

2 tsp tomato purée (no citric acid)
150ml/¼ pint/⅔ cup filtered water
1 small onion, chopped
200g/7oz can tuna in brine, drained
Pinch dried oregano

Mix the tomato purée with the water in a saucepan. Add the onion and cook gently for a few minutes till soft. Flake the tuna and add it to the mixture. Stir, add oregano, and continue cooking till thoroughly heated and the liquid has reduced a little.

** Tuna Risotto

GLUTEN-FREE

This is a delicious meal which I enjoyed when I was on a lecture-tour in Dubai; it seemed to have been 'knocked up' by my hostess in no time at all, and was obviously equally enjoyed by her husband and teenage family. Why not try it on yours?

1 onion, chopped
1 clove garlic, crushed
1 tbsp extra virgin olive oil
3 carrots, peeled and sliced
1 small courgette (zucchini), sliced
2 handfuls frozen peas, sugar-free
1 large can tuna in brine, drained and chopped
1½ large cups cooked brown rice
1 tbsp fresh parsley, chopped
Freshly ground black pepper

Soften onion and garlic in oil and add the carrots and courgette (zucchini). Cook gently with lid on until soft, stirring from time to time. Add frozen peas and cook until thawed. Add tuna, rice, parsley and black pepper and heat through. Serve with a salad or a green vegetable.

White Fish

The following recipes show basic ways for grilling and baking white fish. You can use any sort and any quantity. If you haven't tried cooking fish in a covered dish in a microwave oven, you will find it does it exceptionally well, retaining all the flavour.

---

* Grilled White Fish

GLUTEN-FREE WITHOUT WHEAT FLAKES

Grilling is suitable for flat fish like plaice or sole. Clean the fish and put it in the grill pan. You can squeeze a lemon over it before cooking, if you like, and top it with some crushed wholewheat flakes – though take care, because they burn easily. There is no need to turn the fish; it will be cooked right through quite quickly.

If you like to make a sauce to pour over it, simply mix tomato purée with yoghurt and lemon juice, and heat gently in a saucepan – quantities will depend on requirements, and you can experiment with how much purée you use depending on how much you like tomato sauce!

---

* Baked White Fish

GLUTEN-FREE

This is suitable for thicker pieces of fish like cod steaks or haddock. Preheat oven to 350°F/180°C/Gas Mark 4. Put fish into a casserole dish with 300ml/½ pint/1⅓ cups unsweetened soya milk, juice of half a lemon and a pinch of dried rosemary. If you like, you can add a few tomatoes, sliced. Cover and cook for about 30 minutes.

---

* Poisson del Mar

GLUTEN-FREE

This recipe has a definite continental flavour and is adapted from the cookbook of a Bible College in France, where a client of mine is based as a missionary.

150g/5oz/⅔ cup unsalted butter (or 5 tbsp extra virgin olive oil)
2 large lemons, squeezed

1 large onion, diced
1 tsp fresh parsley, chopped
Freshly ground black pepper
Cod, haddock or halibut steaks, etc.

Preheat oven to 350°F/180°C/Gas Mark 4. Melt the butter (or warm the oil) and mix with lemon juice and diced onion. Add chopped parsley and a shake of pepper. Pour sauce over fish in an oiled or buttered dish. Bake for 25–30 minutes. Serve with brown rice. This recipe is high in fat but its 'richness' is counteracted by the large amount of lemon juice.

** Philippine Fish

GLUTEN-FREE

Here is another recipe with a foreign flavour. The following ingredients serve up to 4, depending on size of squash.

1 squash (butternut, acorn)
Freshly ground black pepper
1 tbsp extra virgin olive oil
1 onion, chopped
1 clove garlic, chopped
25g/1oz/1-inch piece fresh ginger, finely shredded
1 portion per person of cod or coley
400ml/¾ pint/2 cups soya milk (or rice milk)

Preheat oven to 400°F/200°C/Gas Mark 6. Cut squash in half and deseed. Season lightly with black pepper and place cut-side down on an oiled baking tray. Bake for 30–60 minutes, depending on size, until tender. In a minimum quantity of olive oil, stir fry the onion, garlic and ginger. Roughly chop the fish and add it to the pan, covering and cooking gently till done. Remove flesh from the cooked squash and mash, adding enough soya milk to make a creamy sauce. Add to the fish mixture and heat through. Serve with brown rice.

---

* Fish Casserole

MAY BE GLUTEN-FREE

For economy, you could try coley. By the time all the flavours are added to the dish, you will hardly know it from the more expensive types of fish.

450g/1lb cod, haddock or coley fillet
1 small green pepper
4 tomatoes
1 medium onion
25g/1oz unsalted butter
225g/8oz/4 cups broccoli, divided into florets
½ tsp paprika
1 tbsp wholemeal flour (or fine maize meal)
150ml/¼ pint/⅔ cup soya milk (or rice milk)
1 tbsp tomato purée (no citric acid)
1 tsp fresh basil (or pinch of dried basil)
1 clove garlic, crushed, or ½ tsp garlic granules
Freshly ground black pepper

Preheat oven to 325°F/160°C/Gas Mark 3. Skin the fish if necessary, and cut into 5cm/2-inch pieces, being careful to remove any remaining bones. Deseed the pepper and roughly chop it, and also chop the tomatoes and onion. In a saucepan, melt the butter and add the onion, pepper and broccoli florets. Stir over a medium heat for 2–3 minutes. Mix in the paprika and flour (or maize meal) and continue to cook for 1 minute, then add the soya milk, tomatoes, tomato purée, basil, garlic and ground pepper. Bring to the boil and pour carefully into a casserole dish. Stir in the fish, cover with a lid and cook in the oven for 30–40 minutes.

** Fish Lasagne

The above recipe could also be used to make a lasagne, though you don't have to include the broccoli unless you wish, and you could include the juice of half a lemon. The oven needs to be rather hotter than for the casserole, so preheat it to 400°F/200°C/Gas Mark 6. When the fish mixture is ready to pour into the casserole dish, first put sheets of precooked wholewheat lasagne into the bottom. Then add one-third of the heated fish mixture, and so on, ending with a layer of pasta. You could arrange sliced tomatoes on top of this and then add a sauce made from 2 eggs and 300ml/½ pint/1⅓ cups natural yoghurt mixed together. Bake for 35–40 minutes.

** Fish Fingers

MAKES ABOUT 8

A 'must' for the children!

1 large fillet plaice or other white fish (you could use a frozen cod steak)
1 medium potato, cooked till still quite firm, and mashed well
1 free-range egg, beaten
25g/1oz wholemeal flour or soda breadcrumbs

Skin the fish and mash it, removing any remaining bones. Mix with the mashed potato and form into fish finger shapes. Brush with beaten egg and coat with flour or bread-crumbs. Grill 7 minutes each side.

---

* Kedgeree

GLUTEN-FREE

Kedgeree has been one of my husband's favourite meals for many years. Our offspring can remember having it as children in seaside holiday cottages whenever it was Daddy's turn to cook! It has the advantage of being able to use absolutely any type of fish at all – baked white fish or a can of salmon or tuna or even frozen prawns. My own preference is for freshly cooked white fish, preferably haddock. You will soon find your own favourite, and it is so easy to make.

450g/1lb baked white fish (or can of tuna or salmon in brine or 225g/8oz/2 cups prawns)
Optional: 125g/4oz/1 scant cup frozen green peas
125g/4oz/⅔ cup brown rice
2 hard-boiled free-range eggs
2 tbsp fresh parsley or chives
Optional: ½ large can sweetcorn (sugar-free)
Segments of organic lemon

Cook the white fish or open and thoroughly drain the can of tuna or salmon or defrost the prawns, if frozen. Cook the green peas, if using. Roughly flake the fish into fairly large pieces. Cook the brown rice (*see page 160*) and when all the water has been taken up, mix in all the other ingredients. Serve with segments of lemon to squeeze over the top – and enjoy it!

* Herrings, Mackerel and Sardines

The fresh oily fish are so easy to cook yet many people seem frightened to try. Ask the fishmonger to cut off the heads and clean the fish, then all you have to do is wash them (and in the case of herrings scrape off the loose scales with a sharp knife; easy but messy), make two or three slits in one side and put them under the grill for about 5 minutes on each side – the larger the fish, the longer it needs, obviously. Alternatively, bake them in the oven with a knob of butter for 20–30 minutes at 375°F/190°C/Gas Mark 5, or give them a few minutes in a covered dish in the microwave (time depends on size and quantity). Serve with wedges of lemon to squeeze over them. If you don't like eating them off the bone (my husband is a dab hand at doing this efficiently!) you can ask the fishmonger to fillet them for you.

Trout and Salmon

I think that trout and salmon are not often recognized as oily fish because they have a more delicate flavour than herrings and sardines. However, they are just as high in essential fatty acids and therefore can be enjoyed on a frequent basis with real benefit.

* Rainbow Trout

GLUTEN-FREE
Ingredients per person:

1 moderate-sized trout
1 spring onion (scallion)
½ clove garlic
15g/½ oz ginger, finely shredded
1 freshly squeezed lemon

Ask the fishmonger to clean the fish – and to cut off the heads if you can't cope with steely eyes looking up at you! Rinse well under a running tap, flushing the insides, and dry well on kitchen paper. Make 2 or 3 diagonal cuts on both sides of the fish and place in a flat-bottomed dish. Mix together all the ingredients for the marinade, spread evenly over the fish, cover the dish and leave for 30 minutes. Cook under a moderate grill. It isn't necessary to turn the fish because they will be cooked right through. Serve with a salad and jacket potato, or green peas and courgettes (zucchini).

---

* Baked Salmon Steaks

GLUTEN-FREE

1 portion fresh salmon steak per person
1 can tomatoes, chopped (no citric acid)
Fresh basil leaves (or 1 tsp dried basil)
Freshly ground black pepper
1 red onion, chopped

Preheat oven to 400°F/200°C/Gas Mark 6. Place salmon in a flat-bottomed oven dish and cover with chopped tomatoes. Add a few basil leaves or sprinkle with dried basil, a little black pepper and the chopped red onion. Put the lid on the dish and bake in the oven for about 20 minutes.

** Grilled Salmon with Lemon and Coriander

MAY BE GLUTEN-FREE

Ingredients per person:

1 fresh salmon fillet or steak, skinned
1 tbsp extra virgin olive oil
Fennel seeds
15g/½ oz unhydrogenated margarine (or ½ tbsp extra virgin olive oil)
½ tbsp flour (wholewheat, rye, potato, gram, rice)
1 organic lemon (juice and grated rind)
Little soya milk (or rice milk)
Fresh coriander, chopped

Cover the grill-pan with foil (makes washing-up easier and stops the pan smelling of fish) and lay the salmon on it. Brush with oil and sprinkle a handful of fennel seeds over. Place under a hot grill and cook till gently browned, then turn and brown the other side. Meanwhile, melt the margarine or warm the oil in a saucepan and add the flour. Cook gently, stirring with a wooden spoon, until blended together and then slowly add the lemon juice and rind. Add the milk, stirring all the time, until you achieve the thickness you require, then add the coriander and cook for a little longer, taking care not to burn the sauce. Serve the fish with sauce poured over and with jacket or new potatoes and vegetables. If the lemon flavour is too sharp, use only half the juice.

Fish Cakes

Here are some recipes for the very useful fish cake; you can eat it at any meal of the day – breakfast, lunch or supper.

* Salmon Fish Cakes

MAY BE GLUTEN-FREE

3 large potatoes, cooked but still firm
400g/14oz can pink or red salmon, drained
Freshly grated nutmeg
Medium or fine oatmeal to coat (or maize flour or brown rice flour)

Mash the potatoes well and flake the salmon, then mix together with nutmeg. Shape into small round cakes and cover in oatmeal or flour. Grill for a few minutes on each side, till slightly brown and heated through.

Variation: Instead of potatoes, use 2 small sweet potatoes and 1 small kabocha squash, diced, steamed and mixed with herbs.

* Fish Cakes

For another easy recipe, using canned pilchards or mackerel, *see page 269*.

Shellfish

It was pointed out by more than one person that in the first edition of this book I made no mention of shellfish, so they assumed it was not 'allowed'. In fact, I did mention prawns as a starter, or appetizer, but the other types of shellfish I'm afraid were simply overlooked, which is a pity because crab or lobster can help to make a meal 'special', as can oysters and mussels.

Smaller shellfish make appetizing snacks; I happen to live by the sea in a place which has a fleet of cockle boats, and many a stroll includes a visit to the cockle sheds to buy a bag of cockles, whelks or winkles. Having always enjoyed them but considered them rather inferior types of shellfish, it was an eye-opener to find them served at a smart fish restaurant in Paris and at a small hotel on the West Coast of Scotland which served magnificent seafood pasta! If you want to experiment with cooking shellfish yourself, you will need the help of a specialist book; you need to do it carefully and it is something I have never tried. However, you can now buy so many interesting things from supermarkets, including mussels with all the instructions on how to cook them, and fishmongers sell cooked crabs, lobsters and prawns, so you really can make quite a lot of use of shellfish to give variety to your diet. It is good quality protein.

Chapter 26

Eggs, Cottage Cheese and Tofu

Eggs, cottage cheese and tofu all have excellent protein value. However, it is suggested that we eat no more than five eggs per week on average because of their high saturated fat content and their reputed effect on cholesterol (although it is now believed that eggs are less harmful than was previously thought to be the case). Their main uses are perhaps as boiled eggs for breakfast or for Sunday tea, as omelettes for lunch or a light meal, and as one of the major constituents of any sort of quiche. If, in addition to these types of meal, you are eating hard-boiled eggs with your packed lunch, making mayonnaise for your salad and putting eggs in your cake or scone recipes, you can see how easy it is to eat a great many eggs without even noticing.

This section includes several recipes for a wide variety of quiches, because they seem to be a firm favourite with many of my clients. If you are eating quite a few eggs in this way, it would probably be as well to limit them in other forms.

Whether or not you can include cottage cheese in your regime depends on whether you have a dairy intolerance and whether your health improves sufficiently whilst having the small amount of lactose contained in cottage cheese. However, provided it is eaten soon after purchase, it does not contain mould like other cheeses, and it is a very beneficial and useful protein food. The vast majority of my clients are able to fight candida whilst including cottage cheese in their diets, so hopefully you will be the same.

Tofu is an excellent food, being a complete vegetable protein. It is soya bean curd with very little flavour of its own and is therefore good to use in savoury dishes – or the fruit dishes which you make for your family and friends. Not many people seem to know what to do with tofu, but I have received a few recipes for it from some of my clients and you will find them in this section.

Let's start by looking at some simple egg dishes. How about poached egg on a lentil burger? *(See page 179.)* It is nourishing, tasty, and – if you have some burgers ready in the freezer – it is quick. Omelettes also are very quick.

Omelettes

* Herb Omelette

GLUTEN-FREE, SERVES 1

Knob of unsalted butter
2 free-range eggs
Freshly ground black pepper
Pinch of mixed dried herbs
1 tomato, sliced
Parsley to decorate

Melt a small knob of butter in an omelette pan over moderate heat. When hot, quickly break the two eggs directly into the pan and stir them with a round-ended knife, mixing the whites with the yolks and continually bringing the sides to the middle as they start to set. When almost set, sprinkle with black pepper and herbs and quickly fold in half. Slide on to a warm plate, put a row of tomato slices along the top and decorate with parsley. Serve with a slice of soda bread.

** Soufflé Omelette

GLUTEN-FREE, SERVES 1 OR 2

2 free-range eggs
2 half eggshells of filtered water
Freshly ground black pepper

Pinch of dried herbs (try basil)
Knob of unsalted butter
1 tomato, sliced
Parsley to decorate

Preheat the grill. Separate the whites of the eggs from the yolks by breaking an egg into a saucer, up-ending an egg cup over the yolk and pouring off the white into a basin. Measure filtered water into 2 half eggshells, add to the egg whites and whisk thoroughly until light and fluffy. Break up the egg yolks with a fork then gently fold them into the whites. Add black pepper and herbs. Melt the butter in an omelette pan over moderate heat; when hot, add the mixture, stirring gently all the time with a round-ended knife, bringing the sides to the middle until the base is set. Finish cooking by standing the omelette pan under the grill, till the omelette is firm but fluffy and light brown on top. Put sliced tomatoes and parsley on top, and serve whole or cut in half, depending on appetite.

---

* Spanish Omelette

GLUTEN-FREE, SERVES 2

4 free-range eggs
Freshly ground black pepper
Dried marjoram
25g/1oz/knob unsalted butter
1 small onion, chopped
1 red pepper, chopped
1 green pepper, chopped
225g/8oz/1½ cups cooked chopped potatoes

Whisk the eggs with a sprinkling of pepper and marjoram. Melt the butter in a frying pan, soften the onion in it then add the red and green peppers and potato. Cook for a few minutes till the peppers are just tender and the potato heated through, then pour on the whisked eggs. Preheat the grill. Cook omelette in the pan until almost set then put under the grill until golden. Cut in half and serve.

---

* Piperade

GLUTEN-FREE, SERVES 2–4

The following recipe is rather like a Spanish omelette, but uses tomatoes rather than potatoes.

1 medium onion, finely chopped
2 cloves garlic, crushed (or 1 tsp garlic granules)
2 tbsp extra virgin olive oil
2 green or red peppers or mixed, deseeded and chopped
4 tomatoes, roughly chopped
6 free-range eggs
Fresh parsley, finely chopped

Soften the onion and garlic in the oil over a gentle heat for 5 minutes, then add the peppers and tomatoes for a further 5 minutes. Beat the eggs in a separate bowl, then pour over the cooked vegetables and mix them in until lightly scrambled. Garnish with parsley. Cut into required number of servings.

Quiches

To make a quiche, first blind-bake a pastry case as explained on page 100. The quantities below are for an 18–20cm/7–8-inch flan tin, but you could increase amounts by half as much again for a 25cm/10-inch tin. If you have used the microwave for blind-baking, you can either use it for finishing the quiche (High for 7–10 minutes), or you can switch now to the conventional oven, in which case preheat it to 400°F/200°C/Gas Mark 6. The first three recipes use leftover chicken and a variety of vegetables; then there are some which use tuna and others which use just vegetables with one of the various 'toppings', each providing good protein value. The topping for a quiche can be either eggs or tofu, both of which can be combined with yoghurt and/or cottage cheese for even greater variety. Once you have made a few quiches using the following recipes, you will soon see that you can have fun experimenting with all sorts of combinations, and you'll be able to make a delicious quiche with almost anything that happens to be available. Most fillings are *, but if you are making the pastry case at the same time, the whole quiche takes ** energy.

* Chicken and Cucumber Quiche

GLUTEN-FREE FILLING

225g/8oz/1½ cups cooked chicken, chopped
3 spring onions (scallions), chopped
½–1 cucumber, depending on size, peeled and diced
300ml/½ pint/1⅓ cups natural yoghurt
2 free-range eggs, beaten
Freshly ground black pepper
Pinch of tarragon

Preheat oven to 400°F/200°C/Gas Mark 6. Put the chicken, onions and cucumber into pastry case. Mix yoghurt, eggs and seasonings and pour on top. Bake for 30 minutes.

** Chicken and Broccoli Quiche

GLUTEN-FREE FILLING

225g/½lb/4 cups broccoli
125g/4oz/½ cup cottage cheese
1 onion, chopped
2 tsp extra virgin olive oil
½ cup cooked chicken, chopped
3 free-range eggs
Soya milk (added to eggs to make up to 300ml/½ pint/1⅓ cups)
1–2 tbsp chopped parsley
Nutmeg or mace
Note: Tofu Topping (*page 216*) may be used instead of eggs and soya milk.

Preheat oven to 400°F/200°C/Gas Mark 6. Break off the broccoli florets, leaving the larger stalks, and steam until tender. Spread cottage cheese over bottom of pastry case. Soften onion for a few minutes in the oil (in a pan over gentle heat or in the microwave) and spread over cottage cheese. Put broccoli into quiche on top of onions. Add chicken pieces. Beat the egg and soya milk together, pour into pastry case, sprinkle with parsley and nutmeg or mace. Bake for 30 minutes.

Erica White's Beat Candida Cookbook

* Chicken and Avocado Quiche

GLUTEN-FREE FILLING

1 medium onion, sliced
25g/1oz unsalted butter
1 ripe avocado
4 free-range eggs (or Tofu Topping, *page 216*)
3 tbsp chopped parsley
Freshly ground black pepper
175g/6oz/1¼ cups cooked chicken, chopped

Preheat oven to 400°F/200°C/Gas Mark 6. Soften the onion in the butter, in microwave or saucepan over gentle heat. Peel, stone and mash the avocado. Beat the eggs with the avocado till smooth, or blend in a liquidizer. Mix in the parsley and pepper. Put the chicken into the pastry case and pour the mixture over. Bake for 30 minutes.

* Cottage Cheese and Spinach Quiche

GLUTEN-FREE FILLING

1 medium onion, chopped
15g/½oz unsalted butter
275g/10oz/5 cups frozen spinach, thawed
2 free-range eggs, beaten
3 tbsp natural yoghurt
100g/4oz/½ cup cottage cheese
Freshly grated nutmeg
Freshly ground black pepper

Preheat oven to 400°F/200°C/Gas Mark 6. Soften onion in butter in a saucepan, add spinach and simmer for 5 minutes. Beat eggs and mix with yoghurt and cottage cheese. Add to spinach mixture, season and pour into pastry case. Bake for 30 minutes.

* Courgette (Zucchini) and Yoghurt Quiche

GLUTEN-FREE FILLING

125g/4oz/1 cup courgettes (zucchini), thinly sliced
1 medium onion, finely chopped
15g/½ oz unsalted butter
300ml/½ pint/1⅓ cups natural yoghurt
2 free-range eggs, beaten
Freshly ground black pepper
Pinch of tarragon

Preheat oven to 400°F/200°C/Gas Mark 6. Steam courgettes (zucchini) for a few minutes till soft, and soften onion in butter for 2 minutes. Mix together and put into pastry case. Mix together the yoghurt, eggs and seasoning and pour onto vegetables. Bake for 30 minutes.

* Sweetcorn Flan

GLUTEN-FREE FILLING

125g/4oz/½ cup cottage cheese
2 free-range eggs, beaten (or Tofu Topping, *page 216*)
Pinch of dried mixed herbs
Freshly ground black pepper
1 small can sweetcorn (sugar-free)

Preheat oven to 400°F/200°C/Gas Mark 6. Push the cottage cheese through a sieve with the back of a wooden spoon. Whisk together with the beaten eggs, herbs and pepper. Put sweetcorn into the pastry case and cover with the mixture. Bake for 30–40 minutes.

* Aubergine (Eggplant) Quiche

GLUTEN-FREE FILLING

½ an aubergine (eggplant), diced
1 medium onion, chopped
2 tsp extra virgin olive oil
3 free-range eggs, beaten (or Tofu Topping, *page 216*)
300ml/½ pint/1⅓ cups soya milk (or rice milk)

Preheat oven to 400°F/200°C/Gas Mark 6. Lightly fry the aubergine (eggplant) and onion in the oil and put into pastry case. Mix the eggs with the soya milk and pour onto vegetables. Bake for 45 minutes, reducing heat to 300°F/150°C/Gas Mark 2 for the last 30 minutes.

* Tuna and Sweetcorn Quiche

GLUTEN-FREE FILLING

1 medium onion, chopped
1 green pepper, deseeded and chopped
1 tbsp extra virgin olive oil
1 small can tuna in brine, drained
Freshly ground black pepper
½ small can sweetcorn (sugar-free)
300ml/½ pint/1⅓ cups natural yoghurt
2 free-range eggs, beaten
Freshly ground black pepper
Pinch of dried oregano

Preheat oven to 400°F/200°C/Gas Mark 6. Soften the onion and green pepper in the oil for a few minutes. Flake the tuna with a fork and mix with the onion and pepper. Spoon the sweetcorn over the top. Mix the yoghurt, eggs, pepper and oregano and pour over the other ingredients. Bake for 30 minutes.

* Tuna and Tomato Quiche

GLUTEN-FREE FILLING

1 large can tuna in brine, drained
1 medium onion, sliced
25g/1oz/knob unsalted butter
175g/6oz/1 cup tomatoes
3 free-range eggs, beaten (or Tofu Topping, *below*)
2 tsp tomato purée (no citric acid)
2 tbsp chopped parsley

Preheat oven to 400°F/200°C/Gas Mark 6. Flake the tuna. Soften the onion in the butter for a few minutes. Thinly slice the tomatoes and spread over the bottom of the pastry case. Next put in the tuna then the softened onions. Beat the eggs with the tomato purée and parsley, then pour the mixture over the other ingredients in the pastry case. Bake for 30 minutes. Serve hot or cold.

* Tofu Quiche Topping

GLUTEN-FREE FILLING

This makes an excellent egg-free topping with any combination of other ingredients.

125g/4oz tofu
1 tsp dried herbs (any) or 1 tbsp chopped fresh herbs
Pinch of turmeric
Water as required

Filling:
175g/6oz any ingredient or combination of ingredients – see previous recipes for ideas.

Preheat oven to 400°F/200°C/Gas Mark 6. Mix all topping ingredients together in a liquidizer, using only enough water to give a thick, creamy consistency. Put the filling into the pastry case then spread the tofu mixture over it. Bake for 30–35 minutes until the topping is set and slightly brown.

Erica White's Beat Candida Cookbook

Tofu

There are other ways of using tofu apart from in quiches. Here are a couple more ideas for you.

** Baked Pasta and Tofu

MAY BE GLUTEN-FREE

Says this client, 'It is particularly yummy served with fresh watercress and other green salad leaves!'

1 packet of firm tofu, cut into medium-sized cubes
2 tbsp extra virgin olive oil
2 tbsp fresh basil, chopped (or ½ tsp dried basil)
Optional: 1 clove garlic, crushed
225g/8oz/2½ cups pasta twirls or shells (wholewheat, corn, buckwheat, brown rice)
1 medium courgette (zucchini), cut into cubes
1 medium yellow pepper, cut into cubes
1 medium can tomatoes, chopped (no citric acid)
2 tbsp tomato purée (no citric acid)

Place the tofu cubes into a bowl with the olive oil and basil (and garlic, if using). Cover and leave in the refrigerator for 30 minutes. Preheat oven to 400°F/200°C/Gas Mark 6 and also boil the pasta. Put the courgette (zucchini) and yellow pepper cubes into a large saucepan with the tofu mixture and fry very gently over a moderate heat, stirring occasionally, for a couple of minutes until the pepper has softened. Add the chopped tomatoes and tomato purée, stirring until the mixture is heated through, then add the cooked pasta, mix carefully and transfer to a shallow oven-proof dish. Bake in centre of oven for approximately 20–25 minutes.

*** Vegetable and Tofu Stew

GLUTEN-FREE

This would be good with either brown rice or a jacket potato, and it strikes me very much as a healthy, filling meal for a man – and yes, the recipe was sent in by one of my male clients. (Just look at all those precisely-calculated lengths of vegetables!) Seriously, though, thank you Robert for showing other men that they really don't have to starve on the anti-candida diet.

1 litre/2 pints/5 cups vegetable stock
1 tbsp tomato purée (no citric acid)
Dried parsley, thyme and rosemary to taste
1 packet tofu, cut into 1 cm/½-inch cubes
3 tbsp extra virgin olive oil
3 sticks celery, cut into 1 cm/½-inch pieces
1 clove garlic, crushed
4 shallots, cut into eighths
2 carrots, cut into 1 cm/½-inch slices
2 parsnips, cut into 1 cm/½-inch slices
1 leek, cut into 1 cm/½-inch slices
½ tbsp fine maize meal

Heat half the stock, mix with tomato purée and herbs and pour over the tofu. Leave whilst preparing the vegetables, which should all be washed, peeled as appropriate and sliced as shown. Drain the tofu, reserving the stock. Now heat the oil in a non-stick pan and fry the tofu for 5–8 minutes until golden brown. Remove from pan and drain on kitchen paper. Add the celery, garlic and shallots to the pan, adding more oil if necessary, cover and cook gently for 3 minutes. Add the unused stock together with carrots, parsnips and leek and cook uncovered for 8–10 minutes. Add to this the first lot of stock together with the tofu, bring to a simmer, cover and cook for 35 minutes. Dissolve the maize meal in 4 tbsp of cold water, add to the pan and stir in carefully, allowing mixture to thicken.

Chapter 27

Ways with Vegetables

The art of cooking vegetables is to cook them as little as possible. One of the best buys you can make is a stainless steel folding steamer which fits into any size saucepan. The water stays below the level of the steamer so that the vegetables remain crisp. Steaming takes no longer than boiling, and the vegetables have a much better colour, texture and flavour as well as retaining many more nutrients. Even so, if you constantly use a narrow range of vegetables cooked in the same way day-in, day-out, they can become extremely boring, so it is good to think of all the different vegetables which can be used and some of the different ways of cooking them – and please read again my comments on page 58 about buying organic produce, if at all possible.

Potatoes

For many people, the potato is a staple part of their diet, being a filler and good accompaniment to most dishes. The trouble with potato is that, if it is overcooked so that it is soft and fluffy, it very quickly converts to glucose once eaten. You need to stop it cooking just at the point when it is cooked but still fairly firm, and at this stage you get the most vitamins and minerals from it. Because of its readiness to turn to glucose, I am rather wary of recipes which call for mashed potato, but provided it started off as a firm cooked potato, I think it is fairly safe to use. You may have noticed that I never use potato flour in a recipe, and this is why. The best way to avoid glucose problems from potato is to make sure that you eat some fibre with it – whole grains or raw salad are fine, and the potato skin itself is very high in fibre but, as already discussed, you need to weigh up the pros and cons about eating it.

I have received quite a few potato recipes from clients, so here are some of them.

* Potato and Parsnip Bake

450g/1lb/3 cups potatoes, scrubbed
450g/1lb/3½ cups parsnips, scrubbed
4 tbsp fresh parsley, chopped
4 tbsp soda breadcrumbs

Preheat oven to 400°F/200°/Gas Mark 6. Cook the potatoes and parsnips in a little filtered water till just done, then mash with a little of the cooking water, adding the parsley. Lightly grease a baking tin (with butter or extra virgin olive oil), put the vegetables in and bake till crispy, 30–40 minutes. Remove from oven, top with breadcrumbs and return to oven to brown.

** Potato and Tomato Bake

GLUTEN-FREE WITHOUT BREADCRUMBS

1 medium onion, chopped
2 tsp extra virgin olive oil
225g/8oz/1 cup tomatoes, skinned and chopped (or tomatoes from a can without the juice)
1 tsp vegetable bouillon, no yeast
4 tbsp fresh parsley, chopped
675–900g/1½–2lb/4–5 cups potatoes, scrubbed, cooked till just done, mashed
Optional: 4 tbsp soda breadcrumbs for topping

Preheat oven to 400°F/200°C/Gas Mark 6. Soften onion in the oil for a few minutes, then add the tomatoes till heated through and soft. Mix all ingredients together, lightly oil a baking tin, put the mixture in and bake till crispy, 30–40 minutes. If desired, top with soda breadcrumbs and brown as in previous recipe.

** Mediterranean Potatoes

GLUTEN-FREE

675g/1½lb/5 cups potatoes
1 tbsp extra virgin olive oil
50g/2oz/¼ cup unsalted butter
1 clove garlic, crushed (or ½ tsp garlic granules)
1 medium onion
1 green pepper, deseeded and sliced
400g/14oz can tomatoes (no citric acid)
1 tsp mixed herbs
Freshly ground black pepper

Scrub potatoes and cut into even-sized pieces. Cook in enough boiling water to cover, 10–15 minutes till just done. Drain and put in a warm dish. Meanwhile, heat the oil and butter in a frying pan, add garlic, onion and pepper and cook for 5 minutes. Add tomatoes and their juice, breaking up the tomatoes, then add the herbs and seasoning. Cook for 10 minutes. Pour the sauce over the potatoes and serve hot.

** Potato Cake

50g/2oz/¼ cup unsalted butter
1 large onion, thinly sliced
1 clove garlic, crushed (or ½ tsp garlic granules)
675g/1½lb/5 cups potatoes, grated
125g/4oz/1 scant cup plain wholemeal flour
1 tsp potassium (or sodium) bicarbonate
Freshly ground black pepper
2 tbsp fresh parsley, chopped
1 large free-range egg, beaten
2 tsp fresh lemon juice

Preheat oven to 350°F/180°C/Gas Mark 4. Melt half the butter and soften the onion and garlic for a few minutes. Add remaining butter, stir till melted. Put the potatoes in a colander and squeeze out any excess moisture. Put them in a bowl with the flour and bicarbonate, add pepper, onion mixture, parsley, egg and lemon juice and mix well together. Grease a 25cm/10-inch flan tin, press in the potato mixture and bake for 1 hour. Serve hot. Can be frozen; open-freeze in wedges then seal in a plastic bag. To reheat, place on a baking sheet and cook at 400°F/200°C/Gas Mark 6 for 15 minutes.

** Spicy Potato and Cauliflower

GLUTEN-FREE

1 medium onion, chopped
2 cloves garlic, crushed (or 1 tsp garlic granules)
1 tbsp extra virgin olive oil
1 tsp ground mace
1½ tsp ground coriander
1½ tsp ground cumin
2 tsp turmeric
225g/½lb/1½ cups potatoes
225g/½lb/2 cups cauliflower
Boiling water to cover

Soften onion and garlic in the oil over a gentle heat for a few minutes. Stir in all the spices and cook for 2 minutes. Scrub potatoes and chop into small pieces. Break cauliflower into small florets. Add to the pan then pour in enough boiling water to cover. Stir regularly and cook till vegetables are just tender.

* Baked Chips

GLUTEN-FREE

Preheat oven to 375°F/190°C/Gas Mark 5. Scrub two potatoes (peel or leave in skins), cut into 12mm/½-inch slices then cut through again to make chips. Arrange in a layer on an oiled or non-stick baking sheet and bake for 40–45 minutes. This is an excellent way of making chips without fat, and there couldn't be an easier way of cooking potatoes – except perhaps baking them whole in their jackets.

* Baked Potato

GLUTEN-FREE

Jacket potatoes are quick and easy in the microwave but you don't get a crispy skin unless you have a combination oven, which is a microwave, grill and conventional oven combined. Otherwise, for a crispy skin you need to use a conventional oven, which takes considerably longer, or else you could speed things up by part-cooking the potato in the microwave and then transferring to the conventional oven set at a high temperature, say 425°F/220°C/Gas Mark 7. A large potato can take 1–1½ hours in the oven, but you could halve this time by giving it 6–10 minutes in the microwave to start with – depending on size, of course. A longer time at a lower temperature (375°/190°C/Gas Mark 5) will give a tougher, crunchier skin.

Scrub the potato well first, then either prick it all over with a fork or else cut a cross in the top, otherwise the potato might burst out of its skin and give you a very messy oven to clean up!

In view of my warnings elsewhere to peel vegetables thickly in order to reduce your intake of pesticides, should I really be suggesting that you eat potato skins? Well, my personal philosophy is that, provided you don't eat them too often, the nutrient and fibre content of potato skins possibly outweighs the risk of pollutants. Obviously, you must make sure that the skin has been very well scrubbed, but then the choice is yours.

There is an endless variety of fillings you can have with a jacket potato: butter or unhydrogenated margarine or sunflower oil; cottage cheese with chives; mashed tuna or pilchards mixed with yoghurt or cottage cheese; mashed beans with tomatoes – in fact any small leftover portion from a previous day's dinner, provided it has been well refrigerated. I'm sure that no-one really needs me to tell them what they can eat with a jacket potato!

Baked Vegetables

Bearing in mind my comments about the pros and cons of eating vegetable skins, most vegetables can be cooked in the oven rather than on top of the stove, which is convenient if you want to put them in and forget about them for a while and know that they'll be ready when you need them. Parsnips can be baked just like potatoes or may be put into a covered oven dish with any other root vegetables and with just a little water so that they steam rather than bake. Adding a little extra virgin olive oil instead of water gives an interesting variation in flavour and also in texture. Try some experiments!

* Baked Courgettes (Zucchini)

GLUTEN-FREE

4 small or 2 large courgettes (zucchini)
6–8 tomatoes, chopped
1 clove garlic, crushed (or ½ tsp garlic granules)
Pinch of oregano
Pinch of basil
Freshly ground black pepper or paprika

Preheat the oven to 375°F/190°C/Gas Mark 5. Cut the courgettes (zucchini) in half lengthways and scoop out the soft central part, then arrange them in a baking dish. Mix all the other ingredients together, add the scooped-out courgette (zucchini), and pour over the courgette (zucchini) 'boats', filling the boat-shapes and allowing to overflow. Bake for 30 minutes.

Mixed Vegetables

The following recipes show some interesting ideas for cooking mixed vegetables. Similar ideas were contributed by several of my clients, showing that this sort of dish is a regular stand-by accompaniment to a main meal.

* Veggie Pile

GLUTEN-FREE

8 sticks celery, chopped
1 large green pepper, deseeded and cut into long slices
1 large red or yellow pepper, deseeded and cut into long slices
2 large courgettes (zucchini), sliced into rounds
Alternatives: sliced white cabbage is good

Put all the vegetables into a large saucepan or wok with a lid, with just a puddle of boiling water in the bottom. Boil fast for no more than four minutes, but take off the lid and stir a few times during cooking. If you need a nutritious fill-up just for yourself, divide the quantities by four and use a small saucepan.

---

* Vegetable Medley with Sauce

MAY BE GLUTEN-FREE

Assorted vegetables, for example:

Cauliflower florets
Broccoli florets
Carrots, thinly sliced
Celery, cut into 2.5cm/1-inch lengths
Courgettes (zucchini), thinly sliced

Cook the vegetables in a small amount of boiling water for 5 minutes (or preferably steam).

---

* Sauce

1 onion, chopped
2 canned tomatoes (no citric acid)
2 tsp extra virgin olive oil
1 tbsp tomato purée (no citric acid)
1 tbsp wholewheat flour (or fine maize meal)
Freshly ground black pepper
Pinch of mixed herbs
150ml/¼ pint/⅔ cup vegetable stock
To decorate: watercress, chopped spring onions (scallions)

Soften the onion and tomatoes in oil for 5 minutes over a gentle heat. Add tomato purée, flour or maize meal, pepper, herbs and stock, mixing well. Simmer for 5 minutes, stirring. Put sauce into a deep dish and serve the vegetables on top, sprinkled with watercress and chopped spring onions (scallions).

* Ratatouille

GLUTEN-FREE

225g/½ lb/2 cups onions, chopped
2 cloves garlic, crushed (or 1 tsp garlic granules)
2 tbsp extra virgin olive oil
450g/1 lb/4 cups courgettes (zucchini), sliced (or marrow)
450g/1 lb/2½ cups tomatoes, peeled and chopped
1 red pepper, deseeded and sliced
Chopped fresh parsley
Freshly ground black pepper

In a large saucepan with a lid, soften the onions and garlic in the oil over a gentle heat for 5 minutes. Add the remaining ingredients and simmer for 30 minutes.

* Vegetable Kebabs

GLUTEN-FREE

Assorted vegetables, for example:
    Courgettes (zucchini)
    Red and green peppers
    Aubergines (eggplants)
    Cauliflower florets
    Small onions or onion slices
    Cherry tomatoes
Extra virgin olive oil to brush

Wash and scrub the vegetables and cut into equal-sized pieces, approximately 6mm/ ¼-inch thick. Thread onto kebab skewers, alternating vegetables and colours. Brush with olive oil and put under a medium grill, turning occasionally and brushing each side with oil, until just tender. Good with a meal that has a brown rice accompaniment.

*** Roasted Vegetable Tarts

Says this client, 'Rather rich – so keep for a special occasion! Use loose-bottomed flan tins. Best to cook vegetables and pastry case separately.' Linda has to use a gluten-free pastry (*see page 102*), but if gluten is not a problem for you, try any of the other pastries on page 99 onwards.

Make pastry using 6 heaped tablespoons of whichever flours you are using, based on your favourite recipe.

** The filling:

GLUTEN-FREE, MAKES 2 TARTS

1 small courgette (zucchini), sliced
1 red, yellow or orange pepper, deseeded and diced
1 small onion or leek, peeled and sliced
1 carrot, peeled and cut into thin strips
1 parsnip, peeled and diced
1 tbsp extra virgin olive oil
1 tsp dried mixed herbs

Preheat oven to 375°F/190°C/Gas Mark 5. Toss prepared vegetables in olive oil – not too much, just a coating. Arrange in roasting tin, sprinkle with herbs and roast in oven for 45 minutes or until tender. Spoon into precooked pastry tarts and serve.

** Mallorca Spinach

GLUTEN-FREE, SERVES 1–4

1 small aubergine (eggplant) cut into 12mm/½-inch slices
1 tbsp extra virgin olive oil
1 medium onion, finely sliced
500g/1lb/9 cups spinach, washed and chopped
1 clove garlic, chopped
1 beef tomato, skinned and chopped
½ cup water
Freshly ground black pepper
Optional: cottage cheese for crumbling on top

Fry the aubergine (eggplant) in the oil until both sides are light- to mid-brown. Set aside. Fry onion gently until soft. Add spinach, garlic, tomato and water. Cover and simmer until almost cooked, stirring occasionally. Add cooked aubergine (eggplant) and heat through. Sprinkle with black pepper and crumble some cottage cheese on top if required. Serve with brown rice.

*** Buckwheat Crêpes with Spinach

GLUTEN-FREE

This client grows her own interesting varieties of vegetables, and I can vouch for the fact that her spinach is delicious. Thank you, Janet!

Crêpes:

75g/3oz/½ cup buckwheat flour
25g/1oz plain wholemeal flour
3 free-range eggs
50g/2oz unsalted butter (or 2 tbsp extra virgin olive oil)
850ml/1½ pints/3¾ pints soya milk (or rice milk)

Sift flours into bowl and make a well in the centre. Break in the eggs and mix. Melt butter gently with some of the soya milk, add rest of the milk then stir gradually into the flour mixture. Leave to rest for 15 minutes. Heat 25cm/10-inch frying pan, rub pan with buttered (or oiled) greaseproof paper and ladle in a small amount of crêpe mixture. Tilt pan so that the bottom is evenly and quickly coated. Pour out any excess and use less next time. Cook over high heat for about 1 minute, flip over with a fish-slice (or toss it!) and cook second side for a shorter time. Add a little water to the remaining batter if consistency seems too thick. If not serving immediately, pile crêpes onto a plate with layers of greaseproof paper between. Any left over may be frozen.

For the spinach filling:

675g/1½lb/12 cups fresh spinach
2 tsp extra virgin olive oil
1 clove garlic, chopped
50g/2oz/⅓ cup pinenut kernels (or sunflower seeds)
½ tsp freshly ground nutmeg
Sprinkling of fresh lemon juice
4 tbsp natural yoghurt

Wash spinach thoroughly and shred coarsely. Heat oil in a large saucepan, add the garlic and stir-fry for a couple of minutes. Add spinach and stir well. Add all remaining ingredients except yoghurt, cover and cook until spinach is just tender. Mix in the yoghurt. Place a portion of the filling in the centre of each crêpe, roll up and place in a hot oven for a few minutes until warmed through. Serve immediately with a salad.

** Carrot and Corn Bake

GLUTEN-FREE

And, finally, a tasty and satisfying vegetable 'filler' to be enjoyed at any meal, on its own or as an accompaniment.

55g/2oz/½ cup chopped onion
55g/2oz/½ cup chopped celery
2 tbsp unhydrogenated margarine
2 tbsp wholemeal flour
230ml/8fl oz/1 cup soya milk (or rice milk)
2 free-range eggs, beaten
1 large can sweetcorn (sugar-free)
255g/9oz/1½ cups shredded carrot

Preheat oven to 350°F/180°C/Gas Mark 4. Sauté onion and celery in the margarine over a low heat until transparent. Stir in the flour and mix well. Add milk slowly, stirring constantly, and cook until thick and smooth. Remove from heat and add beaten eggs, sweetcorn and shredded carrot, mixing well. Pour into a greased oven dish and bake for about 1 hour, until a knife in the centre comes out clean.

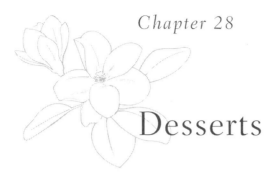

Chapter 28

Desserts

Yoghurt

For people who are not milk-intolerant, low-fat natural yoghurt made from cow's milk is the easiest dessert available. Obviously, you should not eat yoghurt which contains any form of sweetening, or which has fruit in it.

It may seem confusing that you are encouraged to eat yoghurt when you are not allowed most other dairy products. This is discussed in some detail on page 43, but the main benefit of natural yoghurt is that it contains bacteria which are helpful in the fight against candida (*see page 44*). Even so, it is still necessary to take supplements to supply beneficial bacteria because not many 'good guys' in yoghurt will actually be able to travel as far as the large intestine and colonize it, although they will be helpful in the upper part of the digestive tract.

People often think that they should only buy yoghurt which states that it is 'live'. In fact, any ordinary yoghurt can be expected to be 'live', provided you eat it before its 'use by' or 'best before' date, because if you use it as a starter for a new batch of yoghurt, it will work. If it was not live, there would be no bacteria in it to turn milk into more yoghurt. Possibly there will be a greater number of live bacteria in the more expensive products but it should not really be necessary for you to have to pay the extra money.

Greek yoghurt has been strained so that it contains less whey, the watery substance which comes from yoghurt if you leave it standing. There are two things to watch out for when buying Greek yoghurt. Very often it is made from full-fat milk rather than low-fat, so it is fine to have it occasionally as a special treat but not good to eat large amounts of it every day. The other point is that, if it is genuinely Greek and has been imported, it will have had to be pasteurized, and in this case it no longer has any live bacteria. Other forms of yoghurt which are not live are those labelled 'sterilized' or UHT; these have been treated to extend their shelf-life.

As a dessert, Greek yoghurt is more satisfactory because not only does it taste thicker and more creamy, with slightly less of a tang, but the fact that it does not produce pools of watery whey means that it stays looking good in the bowl. You can make it yourself, either from bought or home-made yoghurt, by straining it over a bowl through butter-muslin or cheesecloth. Leave it overnight, perhaps hanging from a tap over the sink, then scrape the yoghurt from the muslin into a basin and keep it in the refrigerator.

There are some people who react badly to cow's milk yoghurt (or to cottage cheese). This is because their immune system is reacting to the protein in the milk, so their reaction is not directly due to candidiasis. It is possible that when the candida has been brought under control and steps taken to help the intestinal lining to become less porous, they will be able to tolerate dairy products once again, but other people are deficient in the enzyme needed to digest milk protein. There are supplements available which supply this enzyme and which can be very helpful in a situation when you are away from home and unable to avoid a certain food containing dairy produce. However, for these people it is best for the time being to learn to live without yoghurt, cheese and butter because they will create an extra burden for the immune system to cope with. An increasing amount of research is being carried out into the many varied enzymes in our bodies and their role in allergy, and this whole area could well be opened up for us in the future.

Some people who react badly to cow's milk yoghurt find that they can tolerate goat's or sheep's milk yoghurt. It is certainly worth experimenting, because yoghurt is an invaluable food for breakfasts, snacks and desserts.

There are various ways of making yoghurt at home, using either an electric yoghurt maker (where little tubs are kept at a constant low heat for 6–8 hours) or a wide-necked vacuum flask. You need a tub of natural yoghurt as a starter for your first batch. After that, you simply save some each time to use as your 'culture' for the next batch, and so on, until the yoghurt starts to become rather 'weak' and you need to start again. It is possible to buy powdered cultures to use instead of shop-bought yoghurt for your first batch. This probably makes a stronger yoghurt which will last through more batches.

* Home-made Natural Yoghurt

1 tbsp skimmed cow's milk powder
600ml/1 pint/2½ cups skimmed cow's milk
2 tbsp natural live yoghurt

Stir the milk powder into the milk in a saucepan, heat to boiling point then leave till lukewarm. Mix a little of the milk with the yoghurt, then add the rest, stirring well. If using a yoghurt-maker, pour into pots and leave 6–8 hours or overnight. If using a vacuum flask, sterilize it first by rinsing with boiling water, allow to cool a few minutes, then pour in the yoghurt mixture, seal, and leave as before. The yoghurt may seem rather runny at first, but cooling it thoroughly in the refrigerator will help it to stiffen.

* Evaporated Milk Yoghurt

I discovered that quite a few people who read this recipe in the first edition of this book had seen that I included evaporated milk and decided that it could therefore be used in other ways – which is most definitely not the case! Please read my lips on this one: evaporated milk is not allowed on the anti-candida diet in any other way except for making yoghurt – which of course is exactly the same rule as for skimmed cow's milk in the first recipe for home-made yoghurt. Both evaporated milk and skimmed milk are just as high in milk sugar, lactose, as any other form of cow's milk but when they are made into yoghurt, the lactose is converted into lactic acid which means it is now beneficial instead of harmful. I have found that using evaporated milk is a particularly fool-proof way of making yoghurt.

1 small carton natural yoghurt
1 large can evaporated milk (full- or low-fat)
2 large cans filtered water (measured in the milk can)

Mix ingredients together thoroughly (an egg-whisk is helpful), pour into tubs for yoghurt-maker or into sterilized vacuum flask as above. Using evaporated milk avoids the need to boil and cool the milk first.

* Goat's Milk, Sheep's Milk or Soya Milk Yoghurts

Any of these can be made by using the same methods as with cow's milk, but in each case you should use the same type of starter yoghurt as the milk you are using; in other words start with goat's yoghurt if you are using goat's milk, etc.

Serving Suggestions

Having made the yoghurt, how can you 'dress it up'? Try 'Yoghurt Surprise' *(see page 68)*. Any combination of seeds, freshly cracked and chopped nuts, lecithin, wheatgerm, or any of the whole-grain cereals can be used. Try crushing up some shredded wheat, or topping the yoghurt with whole puffed rice or puffed wheat cereals. You could crumble up a rice cake or add some popcorn *(see page 114)*. Different textures make it more interesting. I personally love the crunchiness of pumpkin seeds or whole puffed rice.

The next two recipes use Greek yoghurt and can be served attractively in small glass dishes. They can also be used as fillers for pancakes or choux pastry buns, the recipes for which follow later *(see pages 235 and 236)*.

* Coconut Yoghurt Dessert

GLUTEN-FREE

450g/1lb Greek yoghurt *(see page 230)*
½–1 tsp natural vanilla essence
4 tbsp desiccated coconut

Cream all ingredients together. Serve in glass dishes, topped with pumpkin seeds to add some crunch, or use as a filler for pancakes or choux buns.

* French Cream Dessert

GLUTEN-FREE

½–1 tsp natural vanilla essence
450g/1lb Greek yoghurt *(see page 230)*
2 free-range eggs, separated, whites only

Stir the vanilla essence into the yoghurt. Whisk the egg whites until stiff, then gradually fold into the yoghurt. Chill. Serve in glass dishes, topped with pumpkin seeds for crunch, or use as a filler for choux buns or pancakes *(see pages 235 and 236)*.

Carob Desserts

Other creamy desserts which can also be used as fillers are made with carob. Carob is a good substitute for chocolate because it does not contain the stimulants, but it is rather sweet and I feel it should be used with caution *(see page 58)*. However, it is certainly helpful in keeping yeasty children happy on the diet, and it can be used occasionally for a special dessert.

** Creamy Carob Dessert

GLUTEN-FREE

3 x 42g/1½oz bars carob confection (dairy-free, sugar-free)
450ml/16fl oz/2 cups soya milk (or rice milk)
½–1 tsp natural vanilla essence
1 tsp agar-agar
8 tbsp cold filtered water

Break up two carob bars into a basin and stand in a saucepan of hot water. Whilst melting, gently heat the soya milk then gradually pour onto the carob, stirring all the time. Add vanilla essence. When mixed together well, remove from heat. Put agar-agar into the cold water in a saucepan and bring to the boil. When dissolved, allow to cool then stir into the carob mixture. Pour through a sieve into a glass bowl or into individual glasses. Chill in refrigerator until set like blancmange then decorate top with grated carob from the other bar. If this mixture is required as a filling, it can be blended in a liquidizer just before use to make it creamy rather than set.

** Carob Mousse

GLUTEN-FREE

2 bars carob confection (dairy-free, sugar-free)
2 tsp unsalted butter
2 large free-range eggs
Optional: few drops of natural vanilla essence

Melt the carob bars in a bowl over a saucepan of boiling water and add the butter. Separate the eggs, beat the yolks with a wooden spoon and add to the melted carob bars, still over the heat, continuing to beat until the mixture thickens. Take off the heat and allow to cool a little. Meanwhile, whisk the egg whites until stiff and fold into the carob mixture. Replace the bowl over the saucepan of boiling water and beat or whisk further until smooth, adding vanilla essence at this stage if desired. Pour into one large serving bowl or small dessert glasses and leave in the refrigerator to set.

Pastry Desserts

So now we come to some of the puddings which require the above fillings to complete them.

*** Choux Pastry

MAY BE WHEAT-FREE

50g/2oz/¼ cup unsalted butter
150ml/¼ pint/⅔ cup filtered water
75g/3oz/½ cup wholemeal flour
25g/1oz/1 tbsp whole rice flour
2 free-range eggs

Variation: Instead of wheat flour, use 40g/1½oz/¼ cup maize meal and 40g/1½oz/¼ cup barley flour.

Preheat oven to 400°F/200°C/Gas Mark 6. Place the butter and water in a saucepan and bring to the boil. Sift and mix the flours together. When butter has melted, add flours quickly and beat hard until mixture makes a ball. Beat the eggs, then beat them into the mixture. Lightly grease a baking tray, then put on teaspoons of the mixture, spaced well apart to allow for rising. Bake for 10 minutes, then increase the heat to 425°F/220°C/Gas Mark 7 for 15–20 minutes. Split the side of each bun with a sharp knife to allow steam to escape, and cool on a wire rack. These buns can be filled with any of the fillings mentioned earlier – Coconut Yoghurt Dessert, French Cream Dessert, Creamy Carob Dessert – and you can even make profiteroles!

*** Profiteroles

16 choux buns, made from previous recipe
225g/8oz French Cream Dessert (see *page 233*)
4 x 42g/1½oz bars carob confection (sugar-free, dairy-free)
3 tbsp filtered water

When the buns are cool, cut them in half with a sharp knife, fill with French Cream Dessert, and join the halves together again. Pile them into a pyramid on a large dish. Break the carob bars into a basin with the water and melt over a saucepan of hot water, stirring till smooth. Pour the carob sauce over the buns, and serve immediately.

Pancakes

There are many different ways of making pancakes and serving them for dessert, when they can be given the fancy name of 'crêpes'! The basic pancake recipe below can also be used for savoury dishes to make a main meal.

** Basic Pancakes

125g/4oz/1 scant cup wholemeal flour

1 free-range egg
300ml/½ pt/1⅓ cups soya milk (or rice milk)
4 tbsp cold filtered water
Unsalted butter or extra virgin olive oil

Sieve the flour into a bowl and make a well in the centre. Lightly beat the egg then pour into the well. With a fork, gradually mix the flour into the egg, and continue mixing while adding the soya milk. When thoroughly mixed, add the water and whisk well with the fork till the batter is like thin cream. Put a heavy frying pan or omelette pan over a high heat and add a small knob of butter or a few drops of oil. As soon as the fat is hot, add 2 tbsp of the batter, tipping the pan about to ensure that the batter covers the base of the pan. Cook until set, then turn with a fish slice (or toss it!) and lightly brown the other side. Slide onto a warmed plate. Melt another knob of butter or oil before cooking the next pancake. You can make pancakes in advance, stack them on a flat plate and wrap in a clean tea towel, then put them in the refrigerator. Next day you can unwrap them, pile them into a deep casserole dish with a lid, and heat through in a warm oven. When ready to serve, put a warm pancake onto a plate, place a spoonful of whichever filling you are using on one half, and fold over; or spread the filling right over the pancake and then fold it into four.

Wheat-free Pancakes

There are many variations on the theme of pancakes, because you can use virtually any of the whole grains, making them suitable for people who need a wheat-free diet, or even a gluten-free diet. Bear in mind that the wheat-substitute flours will often give rather thicker batters and therefore make heavier pancakes.

** Buckwheat Pancakes

GLUTEN-FREE

Substitute wholemeal flour in the previous recipe with buckwheat or, if wheat is not a problem, use half and half.

** Oat Pancakes

125g/4oz/1½ cups porridge oats or oatmeal
2 free range eggs, separated, whites only lightly beaten
300ml/10fl oz/1⅓ cups soya milk (or rice milk)

Follow instructions for Basic Pancakes, beating well with a wooden spoon or placing all ingredients in a food processor or blender. Oat pancakes might take slightly longer to cook than wheat flour pancakes.

** Rice Flour Pancakes

GLUTEN-FREE

Substitute brown rice flour for wholemeal flour in basic recipe.

** Carob Pancakes

Substitute 25g/1oz/¼ cup of carob powder for 25g/1oz/¼ cup of wholemeal flour in the basic recipe. Sift flour and carob together and blend well.

** American Pancakes

1 free range egg
230ml/8fl oz/1 cup natural yoghurt
1 tbsp fresh lemon juice
2 tbsp extra virgin olive oil
140g/5oz/1 cup wholemeal flour
1 tsp potassium (or sodium) bicarbonate
Filtered water to mix

This mixture is very easily made by putting all ingredients together into a food processor. Otherwise, beat the egg, then add the yoghurt, lemon juice and olive oil, continuing to beat. Sift the flour and bicarbonate powder and stir into the mixture, adding sufficient water to give a thick but liquid consistency. Heat a griddle or a heavy-based frying pan, without oil. Drop spoonfuls of the mixture into the pan in smallish rounds, allowing room to spread. When the edges look done and bubbles pop up on the surface, they are ready to turn and cook for a further minute or two. These may be spread with Lemon Curd (*see page 109*) and used as a dessert or tea-time treat, or they may be used with a savoury spread (*see pages 106–9*).

---

* Lemon and Coconut Sauce

Possibly the flavour we most associate with pancakes is lemon. In my family tradition, at least, lemon pancakes were always a tea-time treat on Shrove Tuesday. Here's a way of recapturing that particular memory.

3 lemons
3 tbsp desiccated coconut (or freshly-grated coconut)

Squeeze the lemons, put the juice in a blender with the coconut and liquidize. Otherwise, just stir well together. Pour mixture onto each pancake, roll up and pour more over the top. Serve while the pancake is still hot.

** Small Cottage Cheese Pancakes

Little cheese pancakes are unusual, and delicious with Coconut Yoghurt Dessert (*page 233*) or French Cream Dessert (*page 233*) spread on top.

40g/1½oz/½ cup wholemeal flour
175g/6oz/¾ cup cottage cheese
25g/1oz/knob unsalted butter, melted
3 free-range eggs, separated
2 tbsp extra virgin olive oil

Sift flour into bowl, add cottage cheese, melted butter and egg yolks. Mix well. Whisk egg whites until stiff, and fold into mixture with a metal spoon. Heat 1 tablespoon of olive oil in a large frying pan and drop 6 separate tablespoonsful of the mixture into the pan, well spaced. Cook over moderate heat for 2–3 minutes, turn over using a spatula or fish slice and cook for a further 2–3 minutes. Remove and keep warm. Repeat with the rest of the mixture.

Cheesecakes

Before I lost my sweet tooth, one of my favourite desserts was cheesecake. I still like the idea of it and it is good to know that there are some pleasant substitutes. Let's look first at some different bases. It's a good idea to use a tin with a press-up bottom, if possible, and it should be lightly wiped round with buttered paper.

* Cheesecake Base 1

Use Basic Shortcrust Pastry mix or Oaty Pastry mix (*see pages 99–100*), blind-baked as on page 100. Alternatively, make the pastry mix but without the added water. Press the mixture firmly, still in its crumb state, into the base of an oiled or buttered tin. Blind-bake in the oven for 15 minutes. If you like a spicy flavour, you can add ½ tsp of ground cinnamon to the flour.

* Cheesecake Base 2

1 tbsp unsalted butter
1 free-range egg
1 tsp fresh lemon juice
125g/4oz/1 scant cup wholemeal flour
½ tsp potassium (or sodium) bicarbonate

Melt butter in a saucepan, beat the egg and add it with the lemon juice to the butter. Sift flour with bicarbonate powder, add to saucepan and mix well. Press dough into the bottom of a buttered dish.

* Cheesecake Base 3

WHEAT-FREE

6 whole rye crispbreads
1 tbsp unsalted butter

Crush the crispbreads in a plastic bag, using a rolling pin. Melt the butter in a saucepan and add the crumbs. Press into the bottom of a buttered tin with a wooden spoon.

** Carob Cheesecake Base

GLUTEN-FREE

175g/6oz unsalted rice cakes
1 x 42g/1½oz bar carob confection (dairy-free, sugar-free)
4 tbsp soya milk (or rice milk)

Crush the rice cakes in a plastic bag, with a rolling pin. Melt the carob in the soya milk in a saucepan and pour over crushed rice cakes. Mix well, press mixture into base of tin, allow to cool then set in the refrigerator. This is good with the carob topping given later (*see page 242*).

Cheesecake Toppings

** Basic Cheesecake Topping

GLUTEN-FREE

450g/1lb/2 cups cottage cheese
600ml/1 pint/2½ cups Greek yoghurt (*see page 230*)
15g/½oz gelatine or agar-agar
4 tbsp water

Press the cottage cheese through a sieve into a bowl, then stir in the yoghurt. Dissolve the gelatine or agar-agar in the water according to instructions on the packet, allow to cool and, when almost set, add to the cheesecake mixture. Pour onto prepared base in tin and set in the refrigerator. This is good with a cinnamon base, as in Cheesecake Base 1.

** Lemon Cheesecake Topping

GLUTEN-FREE

450g/1lb/2 cups cottage cheese
2 free-range eggs, separated
Juice of ½ lemon

Preheat oven to 350°F/180°C/Gas Mark 4. Mix together the cheese, egg yolks and lemon juice. Whisk the egg whites till stiff, fold into mixture with metal spoon. Pour onto prepared base in tin, and bake for 40–45 minutes till slightly brown. Allow to cool. May be chilled in refrigerator or served at room temperature.

** Carob Cheesecake Topping

GLUTEN-FREE

225g/8oz/1 cup cottage cheese
15g/½oz gelatine or agar-agar
4 tbsp water
1 x 42g/1½oz bar carob confection (dairy-free, sugar-free)

Press the cottage cheese through a sieve into a bowl. Dissolve the gelatine or agar-agar in the water according to instructions on the packet. Allow to cool. Grate the carob bar and keep some aside for decorating. When gelatine is almost set, stir into cottage cheese and then stir in most of the grated carob. Pour onto the prepared base in the tin, then put in refrigerator to chill. When set, decorate with remaining grated carob.

Erica White's Beat Candida Cookbook

Everyday Puddings

There are some rather more everyday types of puddings you can have, like rice pudding, semolina, sago and bread-and-butter pudding. Let's look at ways of making these.

** Rice Pudding 1

GLUTEN-FREE

600ml/1 pint/2½ cups soya milk (or rice milk)
225g/8oz/1 cup brown rice
1 free-range egg, beaten
½ tsp ground cinnamon
¼ whole nutmeg, grated
150ml/¼ pint/⅔ cup plain yoghurt

Bring the soya milk to the boil in a thick saucepan and stir in the rice. Put on the lid and cook over a very low heat for about 45 minutes till the rice is soft. (Mind it doesn't boil over, and be prepared to add more soya milk if it gets too dry.) Preheat the oven to 350°F/180°C/Gas Mark 4 and butter a casserole dish. Remove the saucepan from the heat, stir in the beaten egg, cinnamon and nutmeg. Pour the pudding into the baking dish and bake for 30 minutes. When you take the pudding from the oven, spread the yoghurt over it. Serve hot or cold.

* Rice Pudding 2

GLUTEN-FREE

125g/4oz/⅔ cup brown rice flakes
500ml/¾ pint/2¼ cups soya milk (or rice milk)
¼ tsp ground cinnamon
½–1 tsp natural vanilla essence
Freshly grated nutmeg

Preheat oven to 375°F/190°C/Gas Mark 5. Butter a casserole dish and put in the rice flakes, soya milk, cinnamon and vanilla essence. Grate nutmeg all over the top. Bake for 1 hour, stirring occasionally.

---

* Ground Rice Pudding

GLUTEN-FREE

600ml/1 pint/2½ cups soya milk (or rice milk)
5 tbsp brown rice flour
½ tsp ground cinnamon
Freshly grated nutmeg

Heat the milk and stir in the rice flour and cinnamon. Continue stirring over a low heat until the pudding thickens, then cook for another 15 minutes, stirring occasionally. Before serving, grate nutmeg on top.

---

* Semolina Pudding

600ml/1 pint/2½ cups soya milk (or rice milk)
6 tbsp wholewheat semolina (from durum wheat)
1 free-range egg
½–1 tsp natural vanilla essence

Preheat oven to 300°F/150°C/Gas Mark 2. Heat the milk and stir in the semolina. Continue stirring over a low heat until the mixture thickens. Whisk the egg and vanilla essence together, then stir into the pudding. Butter a casserole dish and pour the pudding into it. Bake for about 30 minutes.

Any of the foregoing everyday puddings are very good baked all day in a slow-cooker, ready for dessert with the evening meal, or equally can be cooked overnight and eaten for breakfast.

---

* Sago or Tapioca Pudding

GLUTEN-FREE

(See Chapter 9, page 67, for recipe.)

* Bread and Butter Pudding

If you have some soda bread which is past its best (dry, but not mouldy!), how about using it up in an old-fashioned bread and butter pudding?

5 slices wholewheat, yeast-free soda bread *(see pages 72–8)*
25g/1oz unsalted butter (or unhydrogenated margarine)
425ml/¾ pint/2 cups soya milk (or rice milk)
2 free-range eggs, lightly beaten
¼ tsp ground cinnamon
Freshly grated nutmeg

Preheat oven to 350°/180°/Gas Mark 4. Butter an oven dish. Spread the slices of bread with butter or margarine, cut them into strips and place in the dish, butter uppermost. Warm the soya milk or rice milk in a saucepan, stir in the eggs and cinnamon. Pour over the bread, sprinkle with nutmeg and allow to stand for about 15 minutes before baking in the oven for 45 minutes.

Lemon and Carrot Crumble

MAY BE GLUTEN-FREE

For many people, fruit crumble is a favourite pudding. This next good idea was sent in by Jonathan, who was obviously determined not to be deprived of something he likes so much!

1 organic lemon
125g/4oz/1 scant cup wholewheat flour (or gluten-free flour, *see below*)
50g/2oz/¼ cup unsalted butter (or 4 tsp unrefined sunflower oil or extra virgin olive oil)
1 carrot

Preheat oven to 350°F/180°C/Gas Mark 4. Scrub the lemon well, then grate the rind into a mixing bowl. Add the flour and butter or oil and rub together to form a crumble. Take off the remaining lemon skin and cut the flesh into small pieces. Grate the carrot and place with the chopped lemon in an oven-proof dish with a small amount of water. Place the crumble topping on top of the lemon and carrot and bake for 30 minutes.

Variations to filling: replace carrot with parsnip, sweet potato or turnip; add desiccated coconut or a little cinnamon or nutmeg.

Variations to topping: add sesame seeds, coarse oatmeal or oatflakes, rice flakes, millet flakes etc. For a gluten-free version, replace wheatflour with brown rice, buckwheat or maize flours.

Steamed Pudding

GLUTEN-FREE, SERVES 1

Who says you can't have pudding at Christmas? This one is light and easy to digest, unlike the conventional Christmas pud.

60g/2½ oz/½ cup brown rice flour
40g/1½ oz/¼ cup maize meal
1 tsp carob powder
1 tsp potassium (or sodium) bicarbonate
1 small carrot, grated
2 tsp fresh lemon juice
30g/1½ oz/scant ¼ cup unhydrogenated margarine
4 tbsp soya milk (or rice milk)
Pinch each of ginger, nutmeg, cinnamon, mace

Mix all dry ingredients together in a bowl, stir in the grated carrot and add the lemon juice. Gently melt the margarine with the milk and stir into the mixture in stages, stopping when the mixture is very soft but not runny. Spoon into a greased pudding basin, cover with greaseproof paper and tie up with muslin. Place the basin in a saucepan with enough water to come two-thirds up the sides of the basin. Boil for 1 hour, topping up with boiling water as necessary, or cook in a steamer for the same time. A slow-cooker is an ideal way of cooking puddings because you can leave it all day or all night and forget about it.

Custards

Of course, what you need with a crumble or a pudding is some custard. Try one of these.

---

* Baked Egg Custard

GLUTEN-FREE

3 free-range eggs, beaten
600ml/1 pint/2½ cups soya milk or rice milk
1–2 tsp natural vanilla essence, according to taste
Freshly grated nutmeg

Preheat oven to 325°F/170°C/Gas Mark 3. Butter an oven-proof dish and put in the beaten eggs. Warm the milk in a saucepan then pour it onto the eggs, stirring thoroughly. Add vanilla essence and sprinkle with nutmeg. Put the dish into the oven, standing it on a baking tray which contains cold water. Bake for 40 minutes or until set.

---

* Vanilla Custard

GLUTEN-FREE

Fine maize meal is the unrefined version of cornflour, which is the basis of the custard powder you can buy, so it gives the right sort of consistency; its yellow colour also helps to give it the appearance you expect of custard.

1 tbsp fine maize meal
300ml/½ pint/1⅓ cups soya milk (or rice milk)
1 free-range egg
½ tsp natural vanilla essence

Mix the fine maize meal with a little soya milk to form a paste, then beat in the egg. Warm the rest of the milk in a saucepan, stir it into the paste, then return the mixture to the saucepan and place over a low heat. Continue to stir (or use a whisk) while the custard thickens, then cook (still stirring) for a minute or two more. Stir in the vanilla essence.

---

* Thin Pouring Custard

GLUTEN-FREE

You can make a thicker custard by doubling the quantity of maize meal used in the previous recipe, or you can make a really thin pouring sauce by excluding maize meal completely, as follows:

150ml/¼ pint/⅔ cup soya milk (or rice milk)
1 free-range egg, beaten
¼ tsp natural vanilla essence

Warm the milk in a saucepan, then stir in the beaten egg. Stir over a very low heat until the custard is slightly thick. Add the vanilla essence.

* Spicy Custard

GLUTEN-FREE, SERVES 1

2 tsp maize flour
1 tsp arrowroot powder
Pinch of cinnamon
Pinch of nutmeg or mace
150ml/¼ pint/⅔ cup soya milk (or rice milk)

Sift maize flour through a fine sieve. Mix well with arrowroot powder and spices. Blend to a paste with a little of the milk, then heat the remaining milk in a small pan until it just comes to the boil. Add to the paste and blend thoroughly. Pour back into pan and bring back to the boil gently, stirring continuously.

After-dinner Treats

* Vanilla Bites

MAY BE WHEAT-FREE

This is a delicious alternative when perhaps you are offering guests some fruit or biscuits and cheese to end a meal. They will probably choose the Vanilla Bites instead! Make them at the last minute so the oatcakes don't go soggy.

1 tsp natural vanilla essence
225g/8oz/1 cup cottage cheese
1 plate of oatcakes *(see pages 94 and 260)*
Pumpkin seeds

Mix the vanilla essence into the cottage cheese and pile onto each oatcake. Sprinkle with pumpkin seeds.

** Carob Madeleines

Make mixture as for Celebration Carob Cake *(see page 89)* but omitting the cinnamon, and put into individual, lightly-greased madeleine tins. Fill half-way up then put in a square of carob bar and fill with the remaining mixture. Bake at 350°F/180°C/Gas Mark 4 for 25 minutes. Serve hot with Greek yoghurt or one of the foregoing custards.

One 'naughty' client sent in the following two recipes for Christmas treats. She assures me she only has one or two a week because of the sweetness of the carob!

* After Dinner Mints

GLUTEN-FREE

1 large bar carob confection (sugar-free, dairy-free)
2 drops pure peppermint oil

Melt the carob bar in a bowl over boiling water. When it is gooey, add the peppermint oil and stir. Drop small blobs from a teaspoon dipped in hot water onto a tray covered with a sheet of greaseproof paper. Allow to cool and put in the refrigerator to help the mints set.

Carob-Coated Nuts

GLUTEN-FREE

Make as After Dinner Mints but, instead of adding peppermint, dip assorted nuts into the melted carob. Arrange on greaseproof paper and allow to set in the refrigerator.

All nuts must of course be freshly cracked. Use pecans, hazelnuts, almonds, walnuts or brazils.

Pies

** Butternut Squash Pies

MAY BE GLUTEN-FREE

Here's a more healthy Christmas treat. These make a great alternative to mince pies.

1 large squash (butternut, acorn)
1 batch of pastry (see *pages 99–101*)

Preheat oven to 350°F/180°C/Gas Mark 4 and cook squash as for Squash Muffins (*see page 98*). Make up the pastry, roll it and cut into rounds with a pastry-cutter, cutting slightly smaller rounds for lids. Put larger rounds into a lightly greased and floured bun tray. When the squash is cooked, put spoonfuls of it into the pastry linings and cover with the pastry lids, pricking once with a sharp fork to allow steam to escape. Bake for 20–25 minutes or until golden. Alternatively, you could line a big pie dish, fill with squash and cover with a pastry lid (pricked all over) and cook for about 40 minutes or until golden.

So, there you have a good range of ideas for desserts, some of them quite special. This is one of the longest sections in the book because so many people despair that there is nothing to eat for a pudding except yoghurt. You can of course ring many changes with the baked soya or rice milk puddings by adding different toppings – sunflower or pumpkin seeds for added crunch, grated carob bar for a treat, or desiccated coconut. And, if you are still finding the diet monotonous, try this Impossible Pie – it couldn't possibly be easier!

* Impossible Pie

4 free-range eggs
115g/4oz/½ cup unhydrogenated margarine
60g/2½oz/½ cup wholewheat flour
1 tsp potassium (or sodium) bicarbonate
2 tsp fresh lemon juice
425ml/15fl oz/2 cups soya milk (or rice milk)
85g/3oz/1 cup desiccated coconut
1 tsp natural vanilla essence

Preheat oven to 350°F/180°C/Gas Mark 4. Place all ingredients into a food processor and blend well. Pour into a buttered 25cm/10-inch pie dish and bake for 1 hour. When it is done, you should find (Where's my faith? You *will* find!) that there is a crust on the bottom, custard in the middle and coconut on top!

An 11-year-old boy, determined to win his battle against ME and asthma, stuck determinedly to the anti-candida diet and had his own favourite pudding. It consisted of a chunk of carrot cake *(see page 85)* with a dollop of sheep's milk yoghurt on top, mashed together with his spoon for several minutes. Invited to lunch one day, I watched his face register sheer delight as he ate it, so I decided to give it a try. I agree with him that it takes a lot of beating!

But what about those people who, as well as being on a yeast-free, sugar-free diet also have to contend with the limitations of gluten intolerance and dairy intolerance? Is there no dessert they can enjoy? Well, a little imagination can work wonders.

Avocado Dessert

GLUTEN-FREE, DAIRY-FREE

This client comments, 'I made up this recipe when I realized that I was never going to have another dessert in my life (because of intolerances to dairy and gluten) unless I became inventive!' Well done, Clare; I'm sure a lot of other people in your situation will really appreciate this recipe. Keep coming up with ideas!

3 large carrots
3 large, ripe avocados
1 organic lemon
1 tsp ground cinnamon
Optional: 3 tbsp desiccated coconut
Few tbsp filtered water (or organic carrot juice, no citric acid)
Sesame seeds (optional)

Peel carrots, chop or grate and put in food processor. Add flesh of avocados, zest and juice of lemon, cinnamon (and coconut if desired) and water and blend until a thick 'fool' consistency is achieved, adding more water if necessary. Carrot juice instead of water gives an interesting variation in flavour. Pour into container with lid and refrigerate. Keeps up to 3 days. May be sprinkled with sesame seeds for variety.

part three:

Helpful Ideas

Packed Lunches for Adults and Children

Bases

Fillings

Savouries

Salad

Carrot, celery or cucumber sticks
Tomatoes (especially cherry tomatoes)
Half an avocado rubbed with lemon juice

Desserts

Natural yoghurt
Natural yoghurt with additions – grated coconut, seeds (sesame, sunflower)

Suggested Menu for a Week of Packed Lunches

Monday
Cold chicken drumstick
Oatcakes or soda bread, spread with unhydrogenated margarine
Tomato and a wedge of cucumber
Small tub natural yoghurt
Slice of carrot cake

Tuesday
Tuna sandwich made with soda bread
Celery sticks
Home-made popcorn
Small tub natural yoghurt with desiccated coconut to sprinkle on top
Piece of carob confection bar (dairy-free, sugar-free)

Wednesday
Slice of sweetcorn flan or pizza scone
Pot of salad (lettuce, cherry tomatoes, cucumber, etc.) with favourite dressing
Small tub natural yoghurt with ground sesame seeds to sprinkle on top
Fairy coconut cake

Thursday
Cornish pasty
Carrot sticks with natural yoghurt and celery dip in a screw-top jar
Half an avocado wiped with lemon juice (and a spoon!)
Carob crunchy bar

Friday

Herby scone with cottage cheese
Pot of beany spread
Celery sticks and wheat crackers to dip in beany spread
Corn crisps
Small tub natural yoghurt with sunflower seeds to sprinkle on top
Slice of carrot cake

Chapter 30

Help for Specific Food Intolerances

The foods allowed in the anti-candida diet are sometimes further limited because one or more of them causes a bad reaction. Finding the culprit takes a certain amount of detective work but it could usually be clarified with a simple pulse test which you can do for yourself *(see page 34)*, or a qualified nutritionist should be able to help you. Once you have discovered the offending food (or foods), you will need to avoid it at least until you have brought the candida under control in order to keep that particular burden off your immune system and allow it to fight more efficiently. In time, it might well be possible to help your intestinal wall become less porous, which will help to prevent food allergens from invading your bloodstream and causing your immune system to react. In addition, with an improved nutritional status which will boost your immune system and improve digestive and enzyme systems, your body might well be able to tolerate certain foods in a way which it couldn't before. It is also possible to take specific enzymes in supplement form to help your body cope with the protein in milk products and the gluten in some grain products. However, it is better at first to avoid these foods in order to allow your immune system to be as unhampered as possible.

Among common offenders are cow's milk, eggs, wheat and the other gluten grains (oats, rye and barley). A few unfortunate people can tolerate no grains or flours at all. The following ideas will help you to cope in these difficult situations.

Egg Intolerance

This presents no problem provided that you can tolerate soya. In most baking recipes requiring an egg, you simply replace it with 2 tablespoons of soya flour. You will possibly need a very little extra water. In quiches or flans, you can use tofu instead of eggs, but again this is a product of soya.

Wheat Intolerance

The next sections give ideas for gluten-free and totally grain-free recipes, and these may be used by those who have simply a wheat intolerance. Just to get you started, here is a recipe for wheat-free oatcakes with some interesting variations.

** Wheat-free Oatcakes

225g/8oz/2½ cups oats
50g/2oz/½ cup soya flour
2 tbsp sesame seeds
3 tbsp extra virgin olive oil
Boiling filtered water to mix

Preheat oven to 400°F/200°C/Gas Mark 6. Combine oats, soya flour and sesame seeds. Rub in the oil. Pour boiling water a little at a time, mixing to obtain a firm dough. Leave for a few moments to cool slightly. Roll out and cut into shapes. Place on a non-stick tray and bake until golden.

Variations:
Add any of the following to the dry ingredients before proceeding as above.

2 tsp mixed spice
2 tsp natural vanilla essence
2 tbsp carob powder
4 tbsp desiccated coconut
2 tsp mixed herbs and 2 tsp paprika

For another oatcake recipe *see pages 79–80*.

If you need to avoid wheat for the time being, you may also use almost any recipe in this book which contains wholewheat or wholemeal flour and exchange the wheat for another grain or combination of grain and non-grain flours. Have fun experimenting; you are almost spoilt for choice! Choose from oatmeal, brown rice flour, rye and barley flours, maize meal, buckwheat, milled millet, soya flour and gram flour (made from chickpeas/garbanzos). You can make good use of oats for breakfast (porridge recipes are on page 65), and you can make Oat Bread (*pages 73 and 76*), Oat and Millet Crumble Toppings (*pages 101–2*), Oaty Scones (*page 94*) and Oat or Buckwheat Pancakes (*pages 237–8*). You can also make pancakes from brown rice flour (*page 238*), and pastry from a mixture of brown rice flour and soya flour (*page 102*) or maize meal and rice flour (*page 256*).

If you live near a good health-food store, you will be able to find several different types of wheat-free pasta sold either as spaghetti or as pasta shapes. These include corn, rice and buckwheat pasta; as I said, you are spoilt for choice! Fillers like organic rice cakes, oat cakes and rye crispbreads are now widely available in supermarkets, so you will soon be wondering how there was ever room for wheat in your diet in the old days!

Look at some of the following gluten-free recipes for more ideas.

Gluten Intolerance

Gluten is a protein found in wheat, oats, rye and barley. Gluten intolerance occurs in varying degrees of severity and, at its most severe, is known as coeliac disease. Coeliacs suffer from severe malabsorption and consequent malnutrition and have to avoid gluten grains absolutely strictly in order to stay well. Lesser degrees of gluten intolerance in unsuspecting sufferers can still cause extremely unpleasant reactions affecting both the digestive tract and overall health, and there is usually great difficulty in maintaining or gaining body weight because of the inability to absorb sufficient nutrients from food.

The following is a helpful index to a selection of recipes appearing in this book which may be used by those wishing or needing to avoid wheat, rye, oats and barley. These are just some of the recipes in which you can use alternative grains. However, there are many other recipes in the book which require no grains at all, so these are fine for a gluten-free regime – they have been marked 'Gluten-free' to help you. A few more gluten-free recipes appear after this index.

Spreads

Sauces and Stuffings

Desserts

More Gluten-free Ideas

** Scone Cakes

GLUTEN-FREE

125g/4oz/1 scant cup brown rice flour
50g/2oz/⅓ cup buckwheat flour

50g/2oz/⅓ cup soya flour

2 tsp potassium (or sodium) bicarbonate

2 tbsp desiccated coconut

2 tbsp rice or soya bran

50g/2oz unsalted butter (or 2 tbsp unrefined sunflower or olive oil)

1 free-range egg

1–2 tsp natural vanilla essence, according to taste

4 tsp fresh lemon juice

Soya milk (or rice milk) to mix

Preheat oven to 450°F/230°C/Gas Mark 8. Mix together all flours, bicarbonate powder, coconut and bran and rub in the fat or oil. Beat the egg and mix in, together with vanilla essence and lemon juice, adding enough soya milk to make a dropping consistency. Put a large teaspoonful into oiled bun tins or fairy cake papers. Bake for 15 minutes. May be used instead of bread, cut and filled with cottage cheese, etc.

** Sweet Potato Scones

GLUTEN-FREE, MAKES 5 LARGE SCONES

1 small, pre-cooked sweet potato

Water or soya milk or rice milk

2 tbsp buckwheat flakes for grinding (or buckwheat flour)

4 tbsp maize flour

2 tbsp brown rice flour

1 tsp potassium (or sodium) bicarbonate

1½ tbsp extra virgin olive oil

15g/½oz unhydrogenated margarine

2 tsp fresh lemon juice

Preheat oven to 450°F/230°C/Gas Mark 8. Blend the cooked sweet potato with a little water (or soya milk or rice milk) to make a soup-like consistency. Grind buckwheat flakes in a coffee-grinder (or use buckwheat flour, but it has a stronger taste) and mix with flours and bicarbonate powder in a mixing bowl. Add olive oil, margarine and lemon juice, and rub into flour mixture until it resembles breadcrumbs. Mix in the sweet potato to bind into a soft dough. Add extra liquid if necessary. Flatten balls of dough onto a

Erica White's Beat Candida Cookbook

floured board and cut into rounds with a pastry cutter, about 2½cm/1-inch high. Bake for 15–20 minutes until the scones are a lovely golden colour and sound hollow if tapped on the base. Don't expect them to rise like wheat scones. Eat as soon as possible or freeze as soon as they are cool.

** Rice Crackers

GLUTEN-FREE

Choose a recipe for oatcakes (*pages 79 and 80*), and replace oats with either brown rice flakes or brown rice flour. Add enough hot water to make a moist dough, then leave it to stand for 5 minutes till the water has been absorbed and the dough has become firm. Use plenty of soya flour when rolling. The crackers are fairly hard and crisp. Try variations as in the Wheat-free Oatcakes recipe (*page 260*).

*** Gluten-free Pastry 2

GLUTEN-FREE, MAKES 2 FLAN CASES *(SEE ALSO PAGE 102)*

3 heaped tbsp maize flour
3 heaped tbsp brown rice flour
½ tsp potassium (or sodium) bicarbonate
1 tbsp unrefined safflower oil (or extra virgin olive oil)
15g/½oz unhydrogenated margarine
Water or soya milk or rice milk to mix
1 tsp fresh lemon juice

Preheat oven to 400°F/200°C/Gas Mark 6. Mix flours and bicarbonate powder in bowl. Stir in oil and margarine. Rub in gently until mixture resembles breadcrumbs. Add water (or soya milk or rice milk) and lemon juice slowly and in stages until mixture binds into a soft dough. It is very easy to make the mixture too wet, so be careful. Roll the pastry carefully between two sheets of greaseproof paper. Peel off top sheet and cut out rounds with a pastry cutter according to the size of your individual flan tins. Slide a round-bladed knife under the pastry round, lift carefully and place in flan tins. It will probably break in places, so just do a plastering job with remaining pastry pieces. Prick base all over with a fork and bake for 20 minutes or until cooked and golden. Spoon in filling straight away. (For example, see Roasted Vegetable Tarts on *page 227*.) It is best to use loose-bottomed individual flan tins.

Grain Intolerance

First thoughts are probably that it is impossible to find anything at all to eat if you have to avoid all grains as well as being on the anti-candida diet! In fact, a lot can be done with soya flour (which is made from a bean), mashed peas or lentils (as in pease pudding, gram flour (made from chickpeas/garbanzos), chestnut flour and potato. As with gluten intolerance, don't forget that the recipes in this section are only those which require an alternative to grains; there are very many recipes in this book which need no grains at all and therefore present no problems for you, such as Baked Beans in Tomato Sauce (*see page 175*).

** Soya Cookies

GRAIN-FREE, GLUTEN-FREE

1 mug soya flour
1 mug chickpea/garbanzo (gram) flour
1 mug ground sesame seeds
2 tsp potassium (or sodium) bicarbonate
2 tbsp extra virgin olive oil
4 tsp fresh lemon juice
Filtered water to mix

Variations:
Add 2 tsp mixed spice or ginger, or ½ mug desiccated coconut, or ½ tsp turmeric, ½ tsp paprika and 1 tsp mixed herbs for savoury crackers.

Preheat oven to 400°F/200°C/Gas Mark 6. Combine dry ingredients. Rub in oil. Add the lemon juice and a little water at a time till you have a soft dough. Roll mixture into little balls the size of a walnut and flatten on a greased baking tray. Alternatively, roll out as pastry using plenty of soya flour and cut out shapes with a pastry cutter or the top of a glass. Bake for 30–40 minutes till golden. As with all recipes using chickpea (garbanzo) flour, they need to be well-cooked in order to lose the beany flavour of the chickpeas (garbanzos).

** Soya Bread

GRAIN-FREE, GLUTEN-FREE

Preheat oven to 400°F/200°C/Gas Mark 6. Use the above ingredients but, once you have reached the dough consistency, add soya milk to mix to a dropping consistency, when the mixture is sticky and falls slowly from a lifted spoon. Pack into a greased loaf tin. Sprinkle with poppy seeds, if desired, and bake for 40 minutes. Alternatively, add less milk so the mixture is more like dough, roll into a large round, cut a cross in the top with a sharp knife and bake for about 30 minutes.

** Pease Pudding Bread

GRAIN-FREE, GLUTEN-FREE

Preheat oven to 400°F/200°C/Gas Mark 6. Use ingredients for Soya Cookies *(page 266)* except replace 1 mug of ground sesame seeds with 1 mug of pease pudding (available in cans from health-food stores and supermarkets, but check labels for unwanted additives). Add enough soya milk to obtain a sticky mixture and bake in a greased loaf tin for 50 minutes. Leave in tin to cool before turning out. It's easier to slice if left for a day.

---

* Potato Bread

GRAIN-FREE, GLUTEN-FREE

This is not really suitable for slicing for sandwiches, etc., but is good if cut thickly and topped with sliced tomatoes and grilled for breakfast.

1 mug mashed cooked potato, including skins
1 mug mashed cooked beans (or canned beans, sugar-free)
1 mug soya flour
2 tbsp unrefined sunflower oil or extra virgin olive oil

Pinch of Lo-Salt, if desired
Soya milk (or rice milk) for mixing

Preheat oven to 375°F/190°C/Gas Mark 5. Stir all ingredients together, adding a little soya milk to help mixture stick together, but don't make too wet. Pack into an oiled loaf tin and bake for 40 minutes.

Breakfast Ideas
Breakfast can seem a particular problem on a no-grain diet, so here are some ideas.

---

* Pease Pudding Slices with Tomato

GRAIN-FREE, GLUTEN-FREE, SERVES 2

1 can pease pudding
1–2 tomatoes, sliced
Freshly ground black pepper

Open both ends of the can and push pease pudding through. Cut into six thick slices. Grill both sides then top with sliced tomatoes and continue to grill until tomatoes soften. Serve sprinkled with pepper.

Alternatively, place sliced pease pudding and tomatoes on a covered plate in the microwave. Don't heat too long unless you like your tomatoes mushy!

---

* Tuna Hash

GRAIN-FREE, GLUTEN-FREE, SERVES 1–2

1 tbsp extra virgin olive oil
1 cold cooked potato, chopped into chunks
1 small can tuna in brine
1 tomato, chopped

Heat oil and lightly fry potato. Add tuna and tomato, heat through and serve.

* Mediterranean Breakfast

GRAIN-FREE, GLUTEN-FREE, SERVES 1

1 tomato
Chunk of cucumber
Chunk of white cabbage
1 hard-boiled egg
1 tbsp pumpkin seeds
1 tbsp sunflower seeds
1 tbsp unrefined sunflower oil

Finely chop tomato, cucumber, cabbage and egg. Toss together with seeds and oil. Serve with Soya Bread (*page 74*).

* Pilchard or Mackerel Fish Cakes

GRAIN-FREE, GLUTEN-FREE, SERVES 1–2

Fish cakes are good hot or cold for any meal, but you possibly hadn't considered them for breakfast. Using canned fish means they are particularly quick and easy to make.

1 can pilchards or mackerel in brine
1 tbsp tomato purée (no citric acid)
1 small onion, finely chopped
½ mug soya flour
1 tsp dried mixed herbs

Drain and mash fish and combine well with all ingredients. Make into burger shapes – 4 large or 6 medium. Grill for 5 minutes each side, or fry in a little olive oil, turning after a few minutes, or bake in preheated oven at 400°F/200°C/Gas Mark 6 for 30 minutes. May be frozen cooked or uncooked.

* Bean Burgers

GRAIN-FREE, GLUTEN-FREE, SERVES 1–2
Use above ingredients but replace fish with 1 can of haricot beans (sugar-free), drained, rinsed and mashed. Combine with all other ingredients, make into burger shapes and cook as above.

Fat Intolerance

Steps can be taken nutritionally to help with fat intolerance. For instance, lecithin granules sprinkled on your food each day will help to emulsify fat in your diet so that it is more easily digested and absorbed. (They might also improve your memory, because they are rich in choline, a precursor of the neurotransmitter acetylcholine.) Taking supplements containing digestive enzymes should also help, particularly if they supply the enzyme lipase.

However, most of us eat too much fat in any case so it is good to consider ways of cutting down or avoiding it. It is quite possible to soften onions in tomato juice, for instance, without using oil, even though many recipes in this book do use it. The Baked Beans on page 147 can just as easily be made without oil. It is also quite possible to make a sauce without butter – see recipes on page 147 (Tomato and Onion Sauce) and 146 (White Sauce). It is also easy to make a salad dressing without oil, using yoghurt (*see page 141*). Eggs are high in fat, so you would do better to use soya flour in your baking (2 tablespoons of soya flour with a little water replace 1 egg), and tofu instead of eggs for quiche toppings.

Unfortunately, soya beans sometimes cause problems because they also contain fat, and you might need to experiment with different types of soya milk to see if one suits you better than another.

You can try making oat cakes without fat, but be prepared for a texture which is rather dry and hard. Fortunately, rice cakes and Ryvita contain no fat.

Yoghurt and cottage cheese are generally available in a low-fat form, and hopefully these should cause no problems.

Many of my clients have found that they can tolerate fat more easily as their general nutrition status improves. One lady could not tolerate oil-based vitamin supplements at first (vitamins A, D and E), but after a few months on her recommended diet with other vitamins, minerals and digestive enzymes, she was able to include them with no problems. So persevere, and don't lose heart!

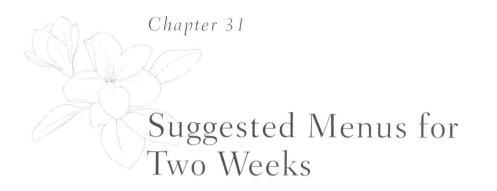

Chapter 31

Suggested Menus for Two Weeks

These ideas do not take account of specific food intolerances, but many can be adapted (see page 59). Numbers shown are page numbers.

WEEK ONE

	SUNDAY	MONDAY	TUESDAY	WEDNESDAY	THURSDAY	FRIDAY	SATURDAY
Breakfast	Tuna Hash 268	Soda bread 73 toasted with seedy butter and tomatoes 69	Creamy Millet 66	Muesli Base 63 with soya milk or natural yoghurt	Scrambled Tofu 70 on soda bread 73	Porridge 65	Boiled egg with rice cakes and margarine
Lunch	Free-range chicken roasted 184 with new potatoes, steamed carrots and courgettes	Mixed raw salad 136 with dressing 138–42 and tinned pilchards	Leek and Potato Soup 129 with soda bread roll 73	Hummus 105 with Oat-cakes 72 and crudités 110	Pizza Scones with raw salad 116	Home-made Baked Beans 175 with soda bread toast and salad 73	Avocado and Tofu Dip 111 with crudités and Sesame Ryvita crackers
Dinner	Wholemeal Scones 92 with cottage cheese and salad. Carrot cake 85	Chicken and cucumber quiche 212 with baked potatoes and steamed carrots	Fish lasagne 202 with salad	Tomato and Tuna Topping 114 with spaghetti or instant wholewheat noodles. Sliced green beans.	Bean and Vegetable Stew 169 with brown rice	Piperade 211 with 'Veggie Pile' 224 and new potatoes	Grilled mackerel and tomatoes with baked chips 222 and baked courgettes 224
Dessert for Lunch or Dinner	Yoghurt Surprise 68	Cheesecake Base 240 and Lemon Topping 242	Coconut Yoghurt Dessert 233	Rice Pudding 243	Vanilla Bites 249	Creamy Carob Dessert 234	Pancakes 236 with French Cream Dessert 233

WEEK TWO

	SUNDAY	MONDAY	TUESDAY	WEDNESDAY	THURSDAY	FRIDAY	SATURDAY
Breakfast	Crunchy Breakfast 64 with soya milk or natural yoghurt	Yoghurt Surprise 68	Scrambled eggs 69 with toasted soda bread 73	Fish Cakes 206	Tomato slices	Creamy Rice 66	Mediterranean Breakfast 269
Lunch	Roast shoulder of lamb 184 with chopped fresh mint, new potatoes, steamed cabbage and baked parsnips	Cold sliced lamb with salad 137 and dressing 138–42	Cream of Tomato Soup 133 with a chunk of soda bread and margarine	Avocado and Lemon Dip 112 with Oatcakes 79 and crudités 110	Seed Rissoles 181 and salad	Chicken Liver Pâté 125 with rice cakes and salad	Bean Burgers 176 with salad
Dinner	Sardine Rolls 118 with salad. Rye slice 91	Seed Loaf 73 with Ratatouille 226	Tuna Bake 198 with Mediterranean potatoes 221	Chicken Kebabs 190 with brown rice and a side salad	Lentil Lasagne 180 with sliced green beans	Aubergine Quiche 215 with baked potatoes and side salad	Grilled plaice 200 with White Sauce 145 and Vegetable Kebabs 226 and a slice of lemon
Desserts for Lunch or Dinner	Carrot and Lemon cake 87 with Pouring Custard 248	Pancakes 238 with Lemon and Coconut Sauce 239	Semolina Pudding 244	Baked Egg Custard 247	Carob Cheesecake 241	Fairy Coconut Cakes 90	Bread and Butter Pudding 245 with Vanilla Custard 247

Chapter 32

Shopping Lists for Suggested Menus

Week 1

Buy organic produce where possible.
Approximate quantities allowing four for each meal.

SUPERMARKET

2 cans tuna in brine
1 can pilchards in tomato
1 can tomatoes (no citric acid)
1 tube tomato purée
2 cans haricot beans (sugar-free)
1 can sweetcorn (sugar-free)
1 tub hummus
4 tubs cottage cheese
2 large tubs natural yoghurt
2 tubs Greek yoghurt
18 free-range eggs
(12 if using soya flour for baking)
225g/½lb unsalted butter
1 packet sesame-coated rye crispbread
1 packet frozen leeks
1 packet frozen cod, haddock or coley
1 free-range chicken
(sodium bicarbonate)

WHOLEFOOD SHOP

Plain wholemeal flour
Brown rice flour
Fine maize meal
Soya flour
Medium oatmeal
Porridge oats
Brown rice
Millet
Wholewheat precooked lasagne
Wholewheat spaghetti
Muesli base (*see page 63*)
Desiccated coconut
2 packets tofu
Extra virgin olive oil
Unrefined sunflower oil
Rice Cakes
Unhydrogenated margarine
Whole puffed rice cereal
4 cartons soya milk or rice milk
Yeast-free stock cubes

Garlic granules
Natural vanilla essence
2 bars carob confection (dairy-
free, sugar-free)
Potassium bicarbonate (?Pharmacy)
(or sodium bicarbonate)
Lo-Salt
Sesame seeds
Pumpkin seeds
Sunflower seeds
Black peppercorns
Agar-agar
Dried oregano
Dried tarragon
Cinnamon sticks
Whole nutmeg
Dried mixed herbs
Dried chives
Ground paprika
Dried basil
Barleycup
Herb teas (?Rooibosch)
Bottled water or filter for water jug

GREENGROCER
12 large potatoes
24 new potatoes
1¾kg/4lb carrots
1kg/2lb courgettes (zucchini)
8 medium onions
4 green peppers
2 red peppers
Salad ingredients
for each day
(*see page 136*)
Vegetables for
crudités (*see page 121*)
20 tomatoes
4 organic lemons
Celery
1 avocado
Cucumber
Spring onions (scallions)
Garlic
Fresh basil
Fresh parsley

Week 2

Please note that you probably have sufficient from last week of items marked '?'.

SUPERMARKET
1 can tuna in brine
1 can pilchards in tomato
1 can sardines in brine
4 cans tomatoes (no citric acid)
? 1 tube tomato purée
1 can haricot beans (sugar-free)
1 can pease pudding
2 tubs cottage cheese
3 large tubs natural yoghurt

WHOLEFOOD SHOP
? Plain wholemeal flour
? Brown rice flour
Bulgar
? Fine maize meal
? Soya flour
? Medium oatmeal
Oatflour
Rye flour
Rye flakes

24 free-range eggs (8 if using tofu for quiche)
and soya flour for baking)
225g/½lb unsalted butter
Frozen chicken livers
Frozen green beans
Frozen (or fresh) plaice
Fairy cake cases
Whole puffed wheat cereal

BUTCHER
1 shoulder of lamb (organic)
450g/1lb chopped chicken

GREENGROCER
9 large potatoes
12 new potatoes
675g/1½lb carrots
1kg/2lb courgettes (zucchini)
12 medium onions
2 green peppers
1 red pepper
Salad ingredients for each day
Vegetables for crudités
1¼kg/2½lb tomatoes
450g/1lb cherry tomatoes
4 organic lemons
Celery
1 avocado
4 aubergines (eggplants)
1 cauliflower
1 white cabbage
450g/1lb parsnips
Garlic
Fresh mint
Fresh basil or dill
Fresh parsley

? Brown rice
Brown lentils
Dried bay leaves
? Wholewheat precooked lasagne
? Wholewheat spaghetti or shells
Wholewheat semolina
? Muesli base (see page 63)
? Extra virgin olive oil
? Unrefined sunflower oil
Wheatgerm
? Rice cakes
Unhydrogenated margarine
? Whole puffed rice cereal
6 cartons soya milk or rice milk
? Natural vanilla essence
2 bars carob confection (dairy-free,
sugar-free)
? Potassium bicarbonate (?pharmacy)
(or sodium bicarbonate)
? Lo-Salt
? Sesame seeds
? Pumpkin seeds
? Sunflower seeds
? Black peppercorns
? Agar-agar
? Cinnamon sticks
? Whole nutmeg
Mixed spice
? Ground paprika
? Dried basil
? Garlic granules
? Desiccated coconut
? Ground cumin
? Ground coriander
? Barleycup
? Herb teas (?Rooibosch)
Bottled water or filter for jug
1 packet tofu

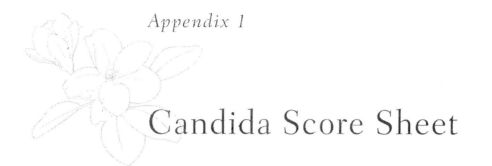

Candida Score Sheet

This candida score will help you to assess the possibility or severity of yeast-related health problems.

Risk Factors

		Points
1) Have you ever taken antibiotics for longer than a month or more than once in a year?	If so, score 5	_____
2) Have you had a high-sugar diet, now or in the past – even as a child? Or have you ever lived through a high level of stress?	If so, score 5	_____
3) Have you ever had a high alcohol intake, or taken drugs?	If so, score 5	_____
4) Have you ever had any steroid treatments – pills, injections, creams, inhalers? (For women, this includes the contraceptive pill or hormone therapy.)	If so, score 10	_____
	Score for Risk Factors	_____

Present Symptoms

Score 1 point per line if any or all of the symptoms are occasional or mild.
Score 2 points per line if any or all of the symptoms are frequent or moderately severe.
Score 3 points per line if any or all of the symptoms are really severe or disabling.

		(Score 1–3)	Points
5)	Depression, anxiety, irritability, mood swings.		_____
6)	Poor memory, lack of concentration, feeling spacey or unreal.		_____
7)	Fatigue, lethargy, feeling drained.		_____
8)	Indigestion, heartburn, food intolerance, bloating, intestinal gas.		_____
9)	Constipation, diarrhoea, irritable bowel syndrome, stomach ache, mucus in stools.		_____
10)	*In women:* Premenstrual syndrome, period pain or irregularities, infertility, endometriosis, loss of sex drive.		_____
11)	*In men:* Prostate problems, infertility, impotence, loss of sex drive.		_____
12)	*In women:* Vaginal burning, itching, discharge.		_____
13)	*In men:* Irritation of groin or genitals.		_____
14)	Muscle aches or weakness, joint pain or stiffness.		_____
15)	Eczema, psoriasis, rashes, itching.		_____
16)	Athlete's foot, ringworm, fungal toenails.		_____
17)	Cravings for sweet foods, chocolate, alcohol, bread.		_____
18)	Sensitivity to perfume, chemical smells, petrol fumes, tobacco smoke.		_____

19) Any symptoms made worse on damp days or in mouldy places.   _____

20) Dizziness, loss of balance, recurrent ear infections, deafness.   _____

21) Insomnia, waking unrefreshed, drowsy during the day, need   _____
    for excessive sleep.

22) Body odour, bad breath.   _____

23) Sores in mouth, sore throat.   _____

24) Nasal congestion, post-nasal drip, sinusitis.   _____

25) Pain or tightness in chest, wheezing or shortness of breath.   _____

26) Urinary frequency, urgency, burning.   _____

27) Spots in front of eyes, burning or watery eyes.   _____

28) Easy bruising, chilliness, cold hands and feet.   _____

29) Headache, migraine.   _____

30) Numbness, burning, tingling, lack of coordination.   _____

31) Irritation around anus.   _____

Score for Present Symptoms (questions 5–31)   _____

Score for Risk Factors (questions 1–4)   _____

Total Score   _____

Total score   75–100   **There is very little doubt that you have yeast infection.**
Total score   50–75   **You very probably have yeast infection.**
Total score   25–50   **You quite possibly have yeast infection.**
Total score   0–25   **Count yourself blessed – but watch your step!**

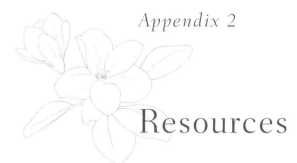

Resources

References and Recommended Reading

Bland, Jeffrey. 'Hidden diseases caused by candida', in *Preventive Medicine*, 3 (4): 12, 1984.

Crook, William G. *The Yeast Connection*, Vintage Books, 1986.

Davis, Adelle. *Let's Get Well*, Unwin Paperbacks, 1985.

Golan, Ralph, M.D. *Optimal Wellness*, Ballantine Books, New York, 1995.

Holford, Patrick. *The Optimum Nutrition Bible*, Piatkus, 1997.

Jacobs, Gill. *Candida albicans: a user's guide to treatment and recovery*, Macdonald Optima, 1994.

McWhirter, Jane. *The Practical Guide to Candida*, All Hallows House Foundation, 1995.

Shaw, William. *Biological Treatments for Autism and PDD*, Health, USA, 1998 (Available from Health Interlink, Interlink House, 1A Crown Street, Redbourn, Herts AL3 7JX.)

Other books by Erica White:

Candida-kuren, published in Norwegian, Ex Libris, Oslo, 1998.

Doughnuts and Temples, Monarch, 1999.

M.E.: Sailing Free, White Publications, 1996.

Erica White is Director of Nutritionhelp Ltd., and members of her team are available for personal or postal nutritional consultations. For details of fees and further information:

Telephone: 00 44 (0) 1702 472085
Fax: 00 44 (0) 1702 471935
e-mail: reception@nutritionhelp.com
Website: http://www.nutritionhelp.com

My favourite recipe, by Emma Watkins (aged 5)

You take a rice cake, and you take some yoghurt,
and you dip your rice cake in your yoghurt.

Useful Addresses of Reputable Supplement Suppliers

UK

BioCare Ltd.
Lakeside
180 Lifford Lane
Kings Norton
Birmingham
B30 3NU
Tel: 44 (0)121 433 3727
Fax: 44 (0)121 433 3879 (General Enquiries)
            433 8705 (Sales)

Nature's Best
1 Lamberts Road
Tunbridge Wells
TN2 3BE
Tel: 44 (0)1892 552117
Fax: 44 (0)1892 515863

USA

Solgar Vitamin and Herb Company
500 Willow Tree Road
Leonia
New Jersey 07605
www.solgar.com

Vital Life
Klaire Laboratories
1573 West Seminole
San Marcos
California 92069
Tel: (760) 744 9680

Thorne Research
25820 Highway 2 West
PO Box 25
Dover
Idaho 83825
Tel: 1 800 228 1966
Fax: (208) 265 2488
E-mail: info@thorne.com
www.thorne.com

How to Learn More About Nutrition

The Institute For Optimum Nutrition runs a three- or four-year Nutrition Consultants Diploma Course. They also run a Homestudy Course, one-day Workshops, Advanced Intensive Courses and a one-year course for medical practitioners and other Health Professionals.

For further news and information on Open Days and Conferences, contact:
I.O.N.
Blades Court
Deodar Road
London
SW15 2NU
England
Tel: 44 (0)181 877 9993

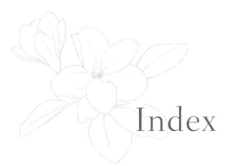

Index

basic white sauce 145–6
batter cakes 90
bean bake 177
bean burgers 176, 270
bean and courgette pie 174
bean paella 173–4
bean sprouts 137
bean and vegetable cobbler 171–2
bean and vegetable pasties 119
bean and vegetable pie 171
bean and vegetable stew 169–71
bean and vegetable stew with dumplings 172
beans 36, 59–60, 166
   dishes 169–80
   types 167–9
beany carrot cake 86
beany salad 142–3
beany spread 107
beany tea cakes 97
beetroot 33
beneficial bacteria 29
beverages 19–20, 45
biscuits 262
black-eyed beans 167
blackcurrant tea loaf 98
Bland, J. 8
blind-baked flan case 100–1
blind-baked quiche 100–1
blood pressure 16, 51
blood sugar 13, 20, 22, 35–7, 48, 52
blood tests 10
body odour 4
body-clock 37
bread 43, 46, 48, 72–8
   gluten-free 262
bread and butter pudding 245
bread rolls 74–5
bread sauce 150–1, 161
breakfast 44, 63–71, 231
   gluten-free 262
   grain intolerance 268–9
breast milk 7–8
breath tests 10

British Medical Association 22
brown lentils 168, 192
buckwheat 35, 162, 165
buckwheat crêpes with spinach 228–9
buckwheat pancakes 237
buffet salads 142–4
bulgar wheat 161
bulimia nervosa 16
butter 34, 44–6, 103, 104, 231, 270
butter beans 167
butternut squash pies 250–1

cakes 85–98, 262
Candida albicans 3–10
   personal history 11–18
   score sheet 3, 10, 277–8
canned beans 59–60
canned fish 197
canned tomatoes 59
cappuccino 159
caprylic acid 14, 16, 18, 26–8
carbohydrates 36, 50
carob 58
carob biscuits 83–4
carob cake 88
carob cheesecake base 241
carob cheesecake topping 242
carob chip cookies 84
carob and coconut shortbread 84
carob cookies 82, 83–4
carob crunchies 91
carob desserts 234–5
carob madeleines 249
carob mousse 233
carob pancakes 238
carob seedy butter 105
carob-coated nuts 250
carrot bread 78
carrot and corn bake 229
carrot and lemon cake 87
carrot and parsnip cake 86
carrot soufflé 125
cauliflower soup 134

demerara 19

depression 7, 14, 16, 25, 35, 40, 51

desserts 230–52, 256, 263

dextrose 19

DHEA 37

diabetes 36

diagnosis 10, 37

Diagnostech laboratory 37

diarrhoea 31

die-off reaction 15–16, 18, 25–7, 31–2, 39–40, 156

diet 18–21, 24–5, 28, 36, 40–52

digestive tract 4, 7, 24, 32–3

dinner parties 53

dips 110–20

dressings 136–44, 270

drinks 45, 154–9

dumplings 172–3

dust 9

earache 7

ears 4

easiest tomato and onion sauce 147

easy oat bread 76

eczema 7, 16, 25, 38

eggplant 34

eggplant quiche 215

eggs 36, 57, 69–70, 208–18, 259–60, 270

eggs with avocado sauce 122

environmental allergies 30

essential fatty acids 21, 51

evaporated milk yoghurt 232

eyes 4

fairy coconut cakes 90-1

falafel 178

families 59

fat-free tomato and onion sauce 147–8

fat-free white sauce 146

fatigue 7, 35

fats 46, 72, 103–4, 270

fermentation 42

fibrositis 11

field beans 167

fillings for packed lunches 255

filter jugs 51, 155

fingernails 22

fish 19, 43, 51, 70, 105, 197–207

fish cakes 206, 269

fish casserole 202

fish fingers 203

fish lasagne 202–3

flageolets 167

flour 56, 72

fluid retention 16, 47

food additives 136

food allergies 4–5, 20, 33-5

food intolerances 259-70

food supplements 18, 21–6, 36

foods to avoid 42–3

foods to enjoy 43–5

four-point plan 18–29

free radicals 104

free-range chickens 183, 184

French cream dessert 233

friendly bacteria 18, 28–9, 38

frozen fish 197

fructose 19, 48, 155

fruit 19, 36, 43, 47–8

fruit teas 45, 51, 155

gadgets 54–5

gallstones 11–12

garbanzo salad 142–3

garbanzos 169

garbanzos in tomato dressing 142

garlic 28–9

garlic mayonnaise 140

ginger cake 87

ginger cookies 81

ginger and walnut cake 88

glandular fever 15

glucose 19, 36, 219

gluten 34, 35

gluten intolerance 259, 261–6

gluten-free pastry 102, 265–6

goat's milk 46, 63, 232
goat's milk yoghurt 233
Golan, R. 8–9, 10
grains 5, 19, 42, 51, 160–3
    food intolerance 266–70
    food intolerances 35–6, 259
gravy 19, 126, 127–8, 187
Great Smokies Laboratory 33
Greek pastitsio 195–6
Greek yoghurt 230-1
green lentils 168
grilled salmon with lemon and coriander
    205–6
grilled white fish 200
grommets 7
ground rice pudding 244
gums 28–9

hair mineral analysis 22
haricot beans 168
hayfever 7
headaches 35, 36, 52
healthy eating guidelines 50–2
herb scones 93–4
herb teas 45, 51, 155, 156
herbs 45, 137
herrings 204
Herxheimer's syndrome 15, 25
Holford, P. 21
home-made natural yoghurt 232
home-made popcorn 114–15
honey 19
hormone treatments 7, 43
hormones 37
hot avocados with dressing 124
hot chocolate 43
hot pilchards and yoghurt 124
house plants 30, 43
household gas 9, 12, 13, 30
hummus 105, 106, 110
hummus dressing 139
hunger 4
hydrogenation 51, 103

hyperactivity 16, 22
hypoglycaemia 35–7

iced teas 157
immune system 4–7, 154, 231
    boosting 15, 21
    food allergies 33–4, 35, 259
    mould 30
    protein 45–6
    smoking 52
    strengthening 28
    toxic metals 22-4
    treatment length 39
    uniqueness 8–9
impossible pie 251
indigestion tablets 22
ingredients 56–9
Institute for Optimum Nutrition 14, 16,
    21–2, 50
insulin 36
intestines 5, 8, 10, 14, 26, 27, 31, 33, 38, 48
irritability 4
irritable bowel syndrome 7, 16

jacket potatoes 223
joints 4, 8
junk food 8, 13, 48

kedgeree 203–4
kidney bean and potato pie 177–8
kidney beans 168

Lactobacillus acidophilus 29
lactose 19, 46–9, 63, 155, 208, 232
lamb 192–6
lamb burgers 194
lamb kebabs 190
lamb lasagne 194
lamb layer pie 193
lasagne 164, 194, 202–3
leaky gut syndrome 9, 31, 33, 35
lecithin granules 270
leek and parsnip soup 131

oaty scones 94
oaty yoghurt soda bread 73
oils 20, 44, 50–1, 57, 103–4
oily fish 197–8, 204
olive oil 104, 164
olive pâté 105
omelettes 209–11
organic foods 58–9, 136–7, 183–4
osteoporosis 24
overweight people 47
oysters 207

packed lunches 78, 255–8
painkillers 20, 43
palpitations 12, 19
pancakes 236–40
pancreas 36
parasites 28, 33
parsnip soup 130
parsnips 223
pasta 164–5
pasta salad 143
pasta sauce 148
pastry 44, 99–102
   gluten-free 262
pastry cookies 82
pastry desserts 235–6
peas 166, 169
pease pudding 70
pease pudding bread 267
pease pudding slices with tomato 268
pepper 58
perfume 9
pesticides 136
Philippine fish 201
pies 250-2
pilchard fish cakes 269
piperade 211
pizza 116
pizza scones 116–17
poisons 8, 9, 22
poisson del mar 200–1
pollution 8-9, 22–3, 136, 155, 197

polyunsaturated fats 103–4
popcorn 114–15
Post-Viral Fatigue (PVF) 9
pot barley 162
potato base 101
potato bread 267–8
potato and broccoli soup 130
potato cake 221–2
potato and parsnip bake 220
potato salad 143–4
potato scones 117
potato soups 128–35
potato and tomato bake 220
potatoes 34, 219–20
poultry 51, 183–96
prawn and avocado salad 123
prawn cocktail 123
prawns 207
pregnancy 7, 11
premenstrual syndrome 16
preservatives 43, 51
pressure cookers 167
pressure-cooked minestrone 133–4
probiotic supplements 28, 29
problems 30–8
profiteroles 236
propolis tincture 29
prostaglandins 51
protein 36, 50–1, 166, 207–8, 231
   food intolerances 259, 261
   immune system 45
Provençal beans 175–6
psoriasis 16
puddings 243–6
puffed rice 63
puffed wheat 63
pulse test 34, 47
pulses 36, 51, 166–82

quiches 208, 211–16
quick chicken pilaff 192
quick home-made baked beans 175
quick spreads 105

quick turkey pilaff 192
quinoa 35, 161

rainbow trout 204–5
raising agents 56–7, 72
ratatouille 226
raw cane sugar 19
recipe use 53–60
red bean dip 114
red bush tea 155
red meat 184, 192
red split lentils 168
refined grains 5, 19, 42
reproductive system 4
resources 279–80
rice 19, 35, 66, 160–1, 165
rice cakes 44, 46, 68, 72, 270
rice and chestnut stuffing 152
rice crackers 265
rice flour pancakes 238
rice milk 44, 46, 63, 155
rice pudding 243–4
roast chicken 185
roast duck 185–6
roast free-range poultry 185–6
roast goose 185–6
roast lamb 184–5
roast turkey 186–7
roasted buckwheat 162
roasted vegetable tarts 227
rock cake scones 95
rooibosch tea 45, 155
root vegetables 137
rye 34, 35, 259, 261
rye groats 162
rye slice 91–2
Ryvitas 44, 270

sage and onion stuffing 152
sago 67
sago breakfast 67
sago pudding 245
salad dressings 104

salads 45, 57, 136–46, 256
salmon 204, 205–6
salmon and cottage cheese dip 113
salmon fish cakes 206
salt 48–9, 51, 58
sardine rolls 118
sardines 204
saturated fats 103–4, 184, 208
sauces 145–52, 225–6, 263
savoury snacks 110, 114–16, 256
schizophrenia 16
scone cakes 264
scones 84, 91–8, 262
scrambled eggs 69–70
scrambled tofu 70
seasoning 58
seed loaf 181–2
seed rissoles 181
seeds 45, 59, 166–82, 181–2
seedy butter 69, 105
seedy cookies 83
seedy tea cakes 97
seedy yoghurt soda bread 73
selenium 24
semolina pudding 244
sesame cookies 81–2
shakiness 4
Shaw, W. 9, 10
sheep's milk 231
sheep's milk yoghurt 233
shellfish 207
shopping lists 55, 274–6
shredded wheat 63
silymarin 31
simple chicken casserole 187
simple dressing 139
sinusitis 11, 25
skin conditions 4, 8
slow-cooker spicy beans 174–5
small cottage cheese pancakes 239–40
smoked fish 19
smoking 24, 52
snacks 116–20